Beyond the Pink Ribbon

WHAT I WISH I KNEW ABOUT BREAST CANCER...
(BEFORE I GOT IT)

By Michele Tripus Orrson

To your Health!

Michele Orrson

Beyond the Pink Ribbon

WHAT I WISH I KNEW ABOUT BREAST CANCER (BEFORE I GOT IT)

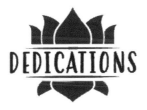

DEDICATIONS

To my Sister Warriors, each with their own stories,
battle scars, and enduring spirits

To Ethan, my joy and motivation for healing my life

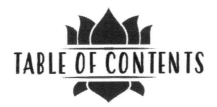

TABLE OF CONTENTS

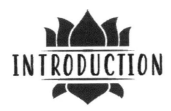

INTRODUCTION

We were headed to China in EPCOT for lunch when the call came. As promised, the radiologist called me on Wednesday during our Disney vacation. "You have invasive lobular carcinoma," she said, as my heart sank. I struggled to hear much beyond that, but I managed to pick up a few words: "Surgeon." "Appointment." "When you return."

And, of course, "Try to enjoy the rest of your vacation."

I wasn't really surprised with the diagnosis because, in my heart of hearts, I already knew. I had spent the past few months wondering what was wrong, and, only five days earlier, I was having my right breast biopsied. That's when I became certain.

But let's back up just a bit, to the fall of 2011. My gynecologist thought he felt a lump in my breast. I had a recent mammogram and it didn't show anything, so he sent me for an ultrasound to be certain. The results of that were definitive: nothing to see here, folks, except a whole bunch of cysts. I always had very cystic breasts and I struggled to know how you could tell a cyst from a tumor. When I did my monthly self-exams, what was I really feeling for anyway?

So, I was sent on my merry way with the usual "see you again next year." In retrospect, I wonder what my diagnosis and treatment would have been if they had told me to come back in six months.

But, during that next year, something was growing. I kept telling myself "Just cysts…just cysts…just cysts." I had done all my due diligence and they found nothing. Carry on. See you in a year.

And yet, it kept growing.

1

Eventually, just a few weeks before my year was up, I made my way back to my gynecologist. I didn't care if it *was* just cysts, but something had to be done. I felt like I had a rock in my breast. A big rock. I couldn't sleep on my right side, I couldn't hug anyone, and the slightest pressure hurt. The nagging in my brain finally pushed me to do something.

My doctor agreed something was amiss. He knew he couldn't send me for another mammogram because the pain of squeezing that rock would have been unbearable. So, I went back for another ultrasound.

This time was different, though. It was late on a Friday afternoon, and the technician took a great deal of time with me. After about 20-30 minutes, she said she needed to get the doctor.

Shit.

Panic started to set in, but I was still holding out hope. The radiologist came in, looked some more, and informed me that I needed to return early the following week for a biopsy.

Shit.

Now with full-blown panic, I informed her that I was leaving the next day for a family vacation in Disney. "Ok," she said, "then we'll have to do it now."

SHIT!

They literally chased people down in the parking lot because it was the end of their shift – on a Friday afternoon – and people were headed home for the weekend. The biopsy was completed and the very comforting doctor said she would call me on Wednesday with results.

She was true to her word when the call came that Wednesday in EPCOT. I remember exactly where we were standing when the phone rang. It's become a tradition that I have my picture taken standing in that same spot every time we return.

We went into the nearest restaurant and ordered lunch while my husband and I did our best to search for whatever information we could on our phones. Mostly I was looking for something that would tell me the likelihood I would die, but that's not really easy to find. What does "invasive" mean? And what the heck is "lobular" carcinoma? Those questions were the tip of the iceberg for all the things I didn't know about breast cancer.

In the end, I decided to follow the doctor's orders and tried to make the most of my vacation. You know, in case it was my last. Plus I didn't want to ruin it for the kids.

Truth be told, I was a lot calmer once I knew for certain, versus just worrying and praying that it wasn't cancer. Now I could take action. It's what I knew how to do. Worrying wasn't productive enough for me. I needed to educate myself. Read. Research. Google. Ask questions. Make decisions. Make changes. I could do something.

There was much to learn about breast cancer, its treatment, and how to be healthy. I just really wished I had known at least some of it before my diagnosis. Not just the BS stuff you get in a pamphlet at the doctor's office, not the pink ribbon awareness crap, but something more: real, valuable information that might have led me to better choices and healthier actions.

Cancer had been present in my life in other ways prior to my breast cancer diagnosis, so you would think I would have paid closer attention to such things. My first husband died of acute lymphoblastic leukemia in 1999, at the age of 43. I watched him battle that horrible disease, and its treatment, for almost three years. It should have been a wake up call. Then, in 2008, I was diagnosed with my own "first" cancer: early stage renal cell carcinoma. I had surgery to remove the tumor and a portion of my kidney, but I failed to learn any lessons from all that. It took my third frolic with cancer to get my act together. Each step of my diagnosis and treatment – from my double mastectomy to chemotherapy, radiation, and beyond – was an opportunity to learn. Cancer was trying to tell me something and it was time to listen.

My journey over the past two decades has led me to this book. My desire is to help others on *their* journeys, and to perhaps even prevent some people from needing to be on this road in the first place. I hope the story of my pain and struggles, my blessings and breakthroughs, the laughter and the tears, will help you in your own quest for cancer prevention and optimal health.

CHAPTER 1

How Aware Are You?

*"Your understanding of what you read and hear is,
to a very large degree, determined by your vocabulary,
so improve your vocabulary daily." ~ Zig Ziglar [1]*

Breast cancer awareness – we've all seen the ubiquitous pink ribbons, most especially during the month of October, plastered on every package known to man. But what level of awareness do those ribbons actually provide? Yes, we're now aware that breast cancer exists. (Is there anyone who doesn't know this yet?) And that it impacts 1 in 8 women. But what else have we learned?

When I received that dreaded call, I realized in that moment just how much I did NOT know. So, in this chapter, I would like to increase your level of awareness. Please indulge me in the vocabulary lesson, but, if you are ever diagnosed, I'd like you to understand what the doctors are saying (or not saying) to you.

ꭓ

Invasive. Lobular. Carcinoma. (ILC)

What does that even mean?

I would quickly learn there is no such thing as just "breast cancer." Rather, there is a wide array of types and variations on a theme. Before I explain some of the nuances, let's define what I had.

Invasive
Adjective. in·va·sive | \in-ˈvā-siv
1: tending to spread especially in a quick or aggressive manner: such as

a) of a nonnative organism: growing and dispersing easily usually to the detriment of native species and ecosystems

b) (1) of cancer cells: tending to infiltrate surrounding healthy tissue

(2) of a pathogenic microorganism or disease: disseminating from a localized area throughout the body [2]

Lobular
Adjective. lob·u·lar | \ˈlä-byə-lər
: of, relating to, affecting, or resembling a lobule [2]

Carcinoma
Noun. car·ci·no·ma | \ˌkär-sə-ˈnō-mə
:a malignant tumor of epithelial origin [2]

Crystal clear now, right?

MayoClinic.org defines Invasive Lobular Carcinoma (ILC) as "a type of breast cancer that begins in the milk-producing glands (lobules) of the breast. Invasive cancer means the cancer cells have broken out of the lobule where they began and have the potential to spread to the lymph nodes and other areas of the body." [3]

ILC has a set of challenges all its own. First, we are always taught to feel for the lumps during our monthly breast self-examinations. Unfortunately, ILC is unlikely to feel like a lump, so you may not find it in a self-exam. ILC feels more like a thickening or hardening of the breast tissue, as was the case for me. I didn't know this, however, since physicians and literature focus on the lumps. There is little awareness that not all breast cancers present in the same manner.

Secondly, ILC doesn't always show up on mammograms. Again, in my case, my regular mammograms never revealed my cancer. My initial ultrasounds did not show it either. Interestingly, when ILC is found, it typically shows up as smaller than it really is. [4] This was also true for me. The initial estimate was that the tumor was "at least 1.8 cm" and, in actuality, it ended up being 8 x 7 x 4.7

cm! That's over 3 inches in diameter! Needless to say, we were all shocked by that! (And no wonder I felt like I had a rock in there!)

Thirdly, if you have dense breast tissue or cystic breasts, finding any type of breast cancer is a bit more challenging because the radiologists need to determine what is cancer and what are cysts. Additionally, the lobes and lobules are a bit deeper in the breast tissue, so it is sometimes in hiding.

ILC only makes up about 15-20 percent of breast cancers. (Yep. I get the weird one.) So what makes up the other 80-85 percent, you may ask? Invasive Ductal Carcinoma, which means that the cancer forms in the milk ducts, which carry the milk from the lobules to the nipple.

While I am not going to cover all of the variations of IDC here, you should know that there are other types: Tubular, Medullary, Mucinous, Papillary, and Cribriform Carcinomas.5 See? Not just one thing.

¨

Other types of breast cancer

In addition to ILC and IDC, there are a number of other types of breast cancer [5]:

- **Ductal Carcinoma In Situ** (DCIS) is non-invasive and found in its original place.

- **Lobular Carcinoma In Situ** (LCIS) is uncommon but is a collective of abnormal cells that may result in ILC in the future. As with ILC, LCIS does not typically show up on a mammogram. Similar to DCIS, In Situ means the cancer is in its original place and hasn't traveled.

- **Inflammatory Breast Cancer,** a rare and aggressive form, is found in 1 percent of breast cancer diagnoses. IBC usually starts with a reddening of the breast rather than a lump.

- **Metastatic Breast Cancer** occurs when the cancer has spread to other parts of the body – typically, to the brain, lungs, liver or bones. This can occur months or years after the original diagnosis. This is also referred to as Stage IV.

- **Paget's Disease of the Nipple** is another rare form of breast cancer impacting a nipple. Usually it is present with another form of breast cancer.

- **Phyllodes Tumors of the Breast** result in leaf-like tumors. These tend to grow quickly but are mostly benign. Some, however, can be malignant.

- **Male Breast Cancer** occurs in less than 1 percent of breast cancers.

Within all of these various types, there are even more breakdowns on the type related to stage, hormone receptors and other variables.

ȣ

Stages of Breast Cancer

Staging doesn't usually happen right away. Often, additional tests are needed, including biopsies and pathological review, and maybe even surgery. I did not find out my staging until after my double mastectomy, when they knew the size of my tumor and the lymph node status.

Stage 0 – Typically referred to as DCIS or LCIS. Found early while the cancer is in its original place.

Stage I – The beginning stage of breast cancer as it starts to invade healthy tissue.

Stage Ia – Cancer has spread to fatty breast tissue.

Stage Ib – Cancer has spread to lymph nodes in small amounts.

Stage II – The cancer is starting to grow larger or spread further.

Stage IIa – This means either there is no tumor or the tumor is under 2cm, but cancer is in the lymph nodes, or the tumor is 2-5cm and not in the lymph nodes. [6]

Stage IIb – The tumor is between 2 and 5 centimeters and cancer has spread to fewer than four lymph nodes or the tumor is larger than 5 cm but has not spread to any lymph nodes. [6]

Stage III – Cancer is more advanced but not yet metastasized to other parts of the body.

Stage IIIa - the cancer is in up to nine of the lymph nodes in the area from your underarm to your collarbone. Or it may have spread to or enlarged the lymph nodes deep in your breast.

Stage IIIb - the tumor has grown into the chest wall or skin around your breast, even if it hasn't spread to the lymph nodes.

Stage IIIc - cancer has been found in 10 or more lymph nodes, or has spread above or below your collarbone

Stage IV – This stage is described as "metastatic," meaning the breast cancer cells have spread beyond the initial area it. Metastasis is most commonly found in the bones, lungs, liver, and brain. [7]

As for me, I was ultimately staged at IIIa due to the size of my tumor and a micro-metastasis in my lymph nodes. A micro-metastasis is small collection of cancer cells that spread from the original tumor. My micro-metastasis was described to me as just some "garbage cells".

ༀ

TNM (Tumor-Node-Metastasis) System for Breast Cancer

Doctors also group cancers by the TNM System. Each letter tells you something about your cancer.

"T" represents your primary tumor. The higher the number, the bigger the mass. Scale of 0-4. At the highest level (there are further subdivisions, T1a for example), T is defined as follows:

TX – Assessment not possible
T0 – No evidence of primary tumor
Tis – Carcinoma in situ
T1 – Tumor ≤ 2.0 cm in greatest dimension
T2 – Tumor > 2.0 cm but ≤ 5.0 cm in greatest dimension
T3 – Tumor > 5.0 cm in greatest dimension
T4 – Tumor of any size but has spread to either the chest wall or breast skin

"N" represents your lymph nodes. Again, a scale of 0-3 and the higher number means more lymph nodes impacted.

NX – Unable to assess lymph nodes
N0 – No lymph node metastasis
N1, N2, N3 – Metastasis in lymph nodes based on how many nodes are affected and how far away the affected nodes are.

"M" stands for metastasis.

MX – indicates they could not measure
M0 – means the cancer has not spread
M1 – reflects distant spread of the cancer [8]

Added to my staging, my diagnosis now looks like this:

Stage IIIa T3N1M0

At the time of reading this on my reports, I had no clue what it meant and, surprisingly, no one explained this TNM system to me. The original staging and TNM assignment does not change, even if your cancer changes. It's intended to evaluate your situation at the time of diagnosis.

ঽ

Tumor Grade

Tumor grade pertains to, as one doctor put it to me, "How ugly the tumor is." It is basically a description of how abnormal the cells look, and their likelihood of spreading. While there are different grading systems for different types of cancer, for breast cancer, the scale is 1-3.

> **Grade I** – cells are mostly normal looking and are usually slow-growing
> **Grade II** – cells are slightly larger than normal, with some odd shapes here and there, growing slightly faster than normal
> **Grade III** – cells are odd shaped and fast growing [9]

My tumor was originally graded as III (poorly differentiated), but was later downgraded to a II after a second review by a cancer expert.

☒

ER, PR, and HER2, Oh My!

This was another grouping of letters that I did not initially comprehend related to my breast cancer subtype. You may hear women say, "I'm triple negative", or "I'm ER/PR positive." When fellow breast cancer survivors talked about this designation, I was a bit lost. I didn't even know I had been tested for this, but it was on my pathology report. My surgeon had indicated that my tumor was estrogen positive (95%) and progesterone positive (35%), and indicated this was all good for treatment purposes.

So what does it all mean?

In a nutshell, ER and PR are related to hormone receptors, meaning that your cancer cells grow in response to the presence of estrogen (ER) and/or progesterone (PR). HER2 is specific to the presence of a protein in the cancer.

About 80 percent of all breast cancers are ER positive and about 65 percent are PR. Only about 20 percent are HER2 positive. What I did learn from my surgeon was the ER and PR positive tumors were "easier" to treat, as they were more responsive to the hormone therapies typically recommended as part of a traditional treatment plan. Examples of these treatments are Tamoxifen,

Arimidex and Femara (which was a real joy ride for me). I will discuss further later on, but I learned the real importance of hormones through all of this.

HER2 positive breast cancers tend to be more aggressive are usually treated with the drug Herceptin.

When your breast cancer is neither ER nor PR positive, AND there is no presence of HER2, it is known as triple-negative. This type of breast cancer tends to return and the risk of relapse is higher in the first few years after treatment. [10]

ጻ

So my final diagnosis looked like this:

Stage IIIa T3N1M0, ER+ PR+ HER2-

Vocabulary lesson over!

CHAPTER 2

Diagnostics

"Luck is not an acceptable substitute for early detection."
~ *Valerie Harper [11]*

In our current medical model, cancer treatment is all about early detection. I know early detection is important, but I feel like this mindset makes the cancer seem inevitable and that we just need to keep looking for it. I'd rather not just sit around and wait for it, but the focus is always on early detection, as opposed to prevention, and so we follow the rules and go for our regular mammograms like the good little girls we are.

I am certainly not suggesting that you shouldn't get mammograms. After all, I went faithfully for decades – they just didn't help me. We all need to make the right decisions for ourselves based on our personal health risks and emotional/mental comfort level.

I am suggesting, however, that you use an abundance of caution, make informed decisions on what diagnostics you have done, and how frequently, based on your risk factors, and recognize mammograms as the imperfect tool they are.

I was one of those people who started mammograms early on due to having fibrocystic breasts (I think I was in my mid-30s). There were some years that I actually went every six months, just to be safe. I remember having a mammogram after my son was born (I was 39). I was told they saw something, and that I needed to immediately have an ultrasound. I sat in that waiting room in tears, in my pink tissue cape, believing that I was about to be diagnosed with cancer and that I would never be able to raise the child for whom I had waited so long. In the end, the "something" was determined to be vascular and life went on. But those minutes of waiting were torturous, and I wonder how many women endure something similar.

As I mentioned in Chapter 1, it's important to remember Invasive Lobular Carcinoma does not always show up on a mammogram. This is because of how the cells grow – in a more linear fashion as opposed to a mass. As such, there may be no lump to feel or see. Additionally, if the ILC does show up on the mammogram, it often appears smaller than it really is. And when you add cysts to the mix, it's even harder to detect. [12]

So while I was a dedicated mammogram-er, it didn't help me find my cancer early. In fact, my gynecologist felt it first, and then follow-up diagnostics indicated it was "nothing" – just cysts. We relied too heavily on those tests and were lulled into a false sense of security. I do wish this were one of the times they told me to come back in six months, rather than a year. Perhaps an earlier diagnosis would have resulted in a lower staging and a less-demanding treatment plan.

Then again, maybe not.

ɤ

Mammography has been scrutinized in recent years for a variety of reasons. First is the exposure to radiation, which can cause DNA damage. While not widespread, some women do get breast cancer from radiation exposure. [13]

There is an ongoing debate about over-diagnosing and over-treating women in situations that very well may never have amounted to anything if left alone. Also, the mortality rate for women who get mammograms is not significantly better than those who do not, especially in younger women. [14] Some countries are even changing their recommendations when it comes to mammograms. [15]

Again, I am not suggesting that you NOT get a mammogram, but rather that you make an informed decision. Ask questions, do your homework, and challenge conventional wisdom if it doesn't feel right for you.

I followed all the rules and ended up with Stage III cancer. On the bright side, my lack of breasts no longer requires me to have my boobs squished into pancakes while zapping them with radiation.

✝

There are other screening options, each with its own set of pros and cons. Often it can be a bit of a fight to get your doctor to request these alternatives, primarily because your insurance company may not want to pay. It never hurts to ask, and I always found it was helpful to enter the conversation armed with data to support your request.

MRI

Magnetic Resonance Imaging (MRI) uses, obviously, a magnetic field and radio waves instead of radiation for imaging. Presently, they are recommended in limited situations due to the cost. [16] After my mammogram and ultrasound, I often wondered if an MRI might have shown my cancer before it got to Stage III. I guess there are a lot of "what-ifs" in our lives.

When I was diagnosed with kidney cancer four years prior to my breast cancer, CT scans were the test of choice. Due to the higher levels of radiation, I was able to convince my urologist to allow me to alternate between MRIs and ultrasounds, knowing that if something odd came up, I'd likely need to have a CT scan. But at least I am not being exposed to additional radiation needlessly.

Ultrasound

Ultrasounds use sound waves instead of radiation to view your breast and allow the radiologist to tell the difference between a tumor and a cyst. This diagnostic tool is usually used in conjunction with other screening, rather than just by itself. If something is seen on a mammogram, often the ultrasound is requested for the purposes of determining if it's a tumor or a cyst, as they present differently. Tumors are solid and cysts are fluid-filled.

Ultrasounds may also be used for younger women who feel a lump. Mammograms are not typically recommended for women under the age of 30 because the breasts contain more milk glands and results are harder to interpret. [17, 18]

Thermogram

Breast thermography uses temperature variations in the breast to identify abnormalities. While thermography is still not widely available or prescribed, it is another tool in the breast cancer tool belt. Like ultrasounds, these are often used in conjunction with other diagnostics, like mammography. [19]

Biopsy

Once something suspicious is found on whatever form(s) of imaging used, the only true way to confirm the presence of cancer is through a biopsy. Guided by imaging, a needle is inserted into your breast to extract one or more pieces of the suspicious lump. [20] They do, gratefully, ensure you are sufficiently numbed before inserting this long, pointy object!

The biopsy process sounded to me like a toy gun snapping each time they took a piece, so while not physically painful, it was a bit unnerving waiting for that sound. They do leave a small metal marker in the location where they did the biopsy for ease of finding it again in future imaging. I was quite bruised afterwards and the area was tender, but generally it was not too painful.

The sample is subsequently sent off for pathology for analysis. My biopsy report read, in part:

Tumor Location:	Right Breast
Tumor Site:	Not Specified
Specimen Type:	Needle Biopsy
Tumor Type:	Invasive Carcinoma
Tumor Size:	At least 1.8 cm
Tumor Grade:	Poorly Differentiated*

And a whole bunch of other terms that I don't understand!

*Poorly differentiated tumors tend to spread more easily and the prognosis is not as good as "well differentiated." Basically, differentiation refers to how closely the cancer cells resemble the surrounding tissue. [21] See Grading in Chapter 1.

Other tests, such as blood work, a bone scan, CT scan and/or PET scan may also be ordered, based on your individual situation. [22]

ℛ

My advice in early detection mode is to do your homework, ask lots of questions, and have a conversation with your doctor around what's best for you. If s/he isn't interested in having that discussion with you (some aren't), then find a new doctor. Ask if the benefits of mammograms outweigh the risks, given family history and health history. Determine which, if any, alternatives might be right for you. Bring facts to the table to challenge conventional wisdom.

And always – *always* listen to your gut.

CHAPTER 3

Risks

"Fate is like a strange, unpopular restaurant filled with odd little waiters who bring you things you never asked for and don't always like."
~ Lemony Snicket [23]

Is cancer something that is fated to happen? Do you think it is destined, no matter what you do?

For some cancers, the answer is "yes". There are genetic factors, to be sure, but it is estimated that only 5-10 percent of all cancers are directly related to genetic mutations. The remaining roughly 90 percent are largely due to lifestyle choices (for example, smoking, poor diet, and excessive sun exposure) and environmental factors (such as radiation, asbestos, and radon). [24]

That 90 percent number truly blew me away and, after my second cancer, I really started taking a hard look at my own behaviors to see if I could figure out why I seemed so "fated" to get cancer. Why was this happening? If it wasn't genetics, what was it, and could I do anything about it?

When I was younger, I had heard about smoking and birth control as being risk factors. Look out if you smoked AND took birth control! You were doomed. But I never heard much else about risk factors.

It turns out there are actually many things that increase your risk of getting breast cancer. Many are also controllable (again, smoking, diet, etc.); others, not so much (for example, age at first period). I think it's important to take some time to review some of the risks. Everyone is different, so maybe 1 or 2 risk factors are enough to result in cancer. For others, they may be able to indulge in a few bad behaviors and never get cancer.

My first husband's oncologist explained it to me this way:

Imagine that there are "switches" in your body, and that you need five switches set to the "on" position for cancer to grow. Some people are born with four of those switches turned on, and so one thing (such as a virus) can flip that last switch, creating the environment for cancer to grow. Other people might be born with only one of those switches set to "on" and, as a result, can smoke and eat cheeseburgers every day with no impact.

When the doctor provided that explanation way back in 1997, it didn't make a lot of sense to me. However, I always remembered the story, and it makes so much more sense to me these decades later. I've also come to realize that healthy lifestyle choices can also turn some of those switches off, reducing your risk. [25] We'll talk about those healthy behaviors in a later chapter, but for now, let's take a look at some of the risk factors for breast cancer. (Note: This is not an exhaustive list.)

The risks bulleted with the checkmarks are all the risk factors that applied to me.

ȣ

Non-Controllable

These are the factors that you really can't help. They aren't behaviors or decisions and "it is what it is." Nonetheless, you should still be aware the risks exist, so you can try your best to mitigate against them. I think of them as incentives for healthy behaviors. [26]

✓ **Gender**
    Breast cancer is 100 times more common in women. Seriously. 100 times. While this book was written primarily with women in mind, it is worth noting that men do, indeed, get breast cancer.

✓ **Age**
As you age, your risk of breast cancer increases. Rates begin to increase at age 40 and are highest in women 70 and older. I had just turned 50 when I was diagnosed, but it had clearly been growing for a number of years.

• **Age at first period**
Women whose periods start earlier than age 12 are at higher risk.

• **Age at menopause**
Women who go through menopause after age 55 are at greater risk.

✓ **Breast density**
The denser your breasts, the greater your risk. Density is determined by the amount of breast and connective tissue compared to fat as seen on your mammogram. So if you aren't sure about this, ask.

• **Genetics**
Most genetic cases of breast cancer are related to the BRCA1 and BRCA2 genetic mutations, accounting for 5-10 percent of breast cancers. I was not tested for this gene since there really was no family history of breast cancer. I did have a genetic consultation to review family history with my parents, but it was determined that a genetic causation was unlikely.

✓ **Height**
Women over 5'3" have a higher risk, by about 10-20 percent. I was 5'6" when I started treatment, and 5'5" when I finished (true story)! I know this for certain, because I was actually measured at my surgeon's office before my surgery and at my one-year mark. I thought it was curious that they did this (none of my other doctors measured my height). I could never find any concrete connection of cancer, or its treatment, to height, but I did find a lot of anecdotes of other women who had lost an inch or two. Their speculation ranged from osteoporosis to chemo to hormone therapies. Again, just one of those weird and curious things.

- **Family History**
  Women who have a "first-degree female" relative (mother, sister, daughter) with breast cancer are almost twice as likely as women without family history. The risk goes even higher if there is more than one family member. Most women with breast cancer do not have family history.

✓ **Personal History of Cancer**
  Women with a prior breast cancer diagnosis are at a higher risk of a new, second primary tumor than women who never had breast cancer before. Additionally, other prior cancers can increase your risk. I was diagnosed with renal cell carcinoma (kidney cancer) in 2008 and it was determined that my two cancers were not related in any way, but it did increase my risk.

Quasi-Controllable

I call these items quasi-controllable since, in some cases, it's based on decision. Other times, there are outside influences.

✓ **Age at first childbirth [26]**
  The older you are when you give birth to your first child, the higher your risk. For some women, it is a choice to delay having children. For others like me, fertility issues were the reason for the delay. I was just six weeks shy of my 39th birthday when I gave birth to my son, even though I had been trying for years to get pregnant.

✓ **Number of childbirths**
  The more children you have, the *lower* your risk. Interestingly, women who do not give birth fall in the middle of risk; they have more risk than those with multiple children, but less risk than those who have their one and only child after 35. Due to my age, prior infertility issues and life situation, I only gave birth to one child.

Controllable (Lifestyle)

✓ **Alcohol Use**
The higher the alcohol usage, the higher the risk. Women who drink 2-3 drinks per day have a 20 percentage higher risk than women who don't drink. Just 2 drinks a day are enough to increase hormone levels in women, increasing their risk along with it.

The National Institutes of Health define low-risk drinking for women as "no more than 3 drinks on any day AND no more than 7 drinks in a week". [27] While I consider myself a social drinker, I'm sure I violated the NIH guidelines more times than I'd like to admit.

✓ **Birth Control Pills [26]**
Current or recent use of birth control pills increases risk. While taking the pill, or shortly after stopping, risk is 20-30 percent higher than for women who never used the pill. Once you stop, over time, the risk reduces. Prior to my diagnosis, I was on birth control pills. And, in fact, I was skipping the placebo week to help with migraines. In retrospect, this was probably not the best idea.

✓ **Weight Gain**
Gaining weight after the age of 18 (yikes, who doesn't do this?), increases breast cancer risk. One study found that gaining just 20 pounds after age 18 increased risk by 15 percent. Women who gained 55 pounds or more had a 45 percent higher risk. I was pretty skinny (around 120 pounds in college) until my mid-20s. At my highest weight (in the 1990s), I was over 170 pounds. So, yeah, that's 50-ish pounds.

✓ **Poor Diet**
Diet is believed to be a factor in cancer initiation and growth. It is believed that as much as 30-40 percent of cancers are related to diet. [28] The Standard American Diet (SAD), complete with its high-fat, high-salt, highly-processed, nutrient-poor foods, contributes to a number of chronic diseases, including cancer. Without the proper nutrients, our bodies become inflamed and cannot adequately fight off disease.

I was definitely a SAD eater. A busy lifestyle led to too many take-out foods (pizza and Chinese were my go-to places), and my cooking repertoire was severely limited. I grew up in a meat and potatoes home and felt that meat needed to be on every plate. My fruit and vegetable intake was insufficient, and whole grains were nowhere to be found. (More on diet in Chapters 8 & 9.)

✓ **Lack of Exercise**
Related to being overweight, people who don't exercise tend to weigh more than those that do. Fat cells make estrogen. More fat cells mean more estrogen and the increased estrogen levels over time increases your risk. I was never a big fan of exercise (I'm still not). This is an area in which I need to make some improvements. I love yoga (which I will do in fits and starts) and will happily walk on a treadmill if I can do something productive at the same time. While I know intellectually all the benefits of exercise, I have an ongoing struggle with making it a priority.

• **Smoking**
Smoking and exposure to secondhand smoke are risk factors for breast cancer, as well as lung cancer, heart disease, and a variety of other illnesses. Smoking also can result in complications during treatment and slow the healing process. If you smoke, the absolute best thing you can do for yourself and your loved ones is to quit. [29, 30]

✓ **Overuse of Antibiotics**
While not widely accepted in the medical field, there is some evidence that overuse of antibiotics can contribute to certain types of cancer. A few studies have been done showing an association of antibiotics use and breast cancer risk. It is believed that the antibiotics affect the immune system, inhibiting it from fighting cancer. [31]

Anecdotally, I can relate to this connection, as someone who probably took a few too many antibiotics over the years. It was a vicious cycle of sinus infections (antibiotic A) followed by UTIs (from antibiotic A resulting in the need for antibiotic B), several times a year. I knew it was bad when we were having septic system issues and the workers who came to fix our problems said they only see this type of bubbling up with "old people who take lots of antibiotics". Yikes! I wasn't old but I confessed to the overuse. The technician didn't believe me, but it was enough for me to realize I needed to stop. Now, I try to never take them.

ℜ

So there you have it – a list of many breast cancer risks. In case you weren't counting, I actually had 13 of the ones I have listed. I know no one wants to think that their behaviors and choices may have contributed to their own disease. Do I blame myself? Do I feel guilty about it? Actually, I don't. What I do feel is hope, because if my behaviors contributed to illness, then I can take control of those behaviors. I can make changes and, perhaps, lead a much healthier life going forward.

It isn't Fate.

It isn't always inevitable.

CHAPTER 4

Treatment & Side Effects: Surgery

"The wound is the place where the Light enters you." ~ Rumi

My treatment plan included surgery, chemotherapy, radiation and hormone therapy; the whole ball of wax – and in that order. As I understand it, this is the most typical sequence: Cut it out, then poison it, radiate it and eliminate any hormones that may have fed your tumor. Sounds positively delightful, doesn't it? There are times when these treatments may be given in a different order; for example, chemotherapy before surgery.

In the next few chapters, I'll discuss my experiences with each treatment option, along with the side effects I encountered and some self-care tips.

ჯ

I met with my surgeon upon returning from Disney. I didn't want to rush into the surgery since school would be starting in the coming weeks and I wanted a smooth transition for my son. My surgery was scheduled for August 31, 2012, and the plan was for removal of my right breast. As the days ticked by, however, something bothered me about this decision, and it had nothing to do with *IF* I should do it.

I was actually uneasy about being asymmetrical. How would I handle having a uni-boob? Would I then feel compelled to go through reconstruction at some point, or always wear a prosthetic, for symmetry? This seemed like a petty concern and I kept trying to brush it off, but it lingered.

Then, when I was having my pre-admission testing done, I had a wonderful conversation with my nurse. She explained to me that she was a 25-year survivor, having had breast cancer in one breast, and then a few years after that, getting it in the other breast. And there it was. The real reason for my concern: getting cancer in the other breast. I just couldn't bear getting cancer a *third* time.

And so, I called my gynecologist (who I love and whose opinion I value greatly) and expressed my desire to have a double mastectomy. He agreed it was probably the right decision for me considering my history. I then consulted with my surgeon, who quickly got approval from the insurance company. I thought I might actually have to fight with them, but apparently "prophylactic" removal of breasts was a common thing. I was actually surprised at how quickly it all transpired, from single to double, from decision to approval. I am grateful for that conversation with the nurse. You never know who is going to be put in your path to help you make the right decisions along the way.

I also opted for no reconstruction. This decision was definitely the right one for *ME*. I think there are many factors that go into the decision-making process and every woman needs to make her own decision. Don't let *ANYONE* force you into a decision. I had several women telling me which reconstruction option I should pick based on their experiences, but I held my ground.

Perhaps if I was younger, or had no prior cancer history, or was a different size/shape, or worked in an industry where my appearance mattered, I might have considered reconstruction. But I was 50 years old, and this was my second cancer. I just wanted it *OUT*. I wanted to get strong, to heal from the surgery, and just get my chemo done. I didn't want to have to worry about expanders and infections and discomfort. I had heard too many stories about reconstruction to be interested. The surgeon always left the option open for me and I could still decide to do it at any point in the future (I won't). In fact, he always told me, "The safest surgery is the one you never have."

I have no regrets about this decision and don't really think about it most days. Yes, I have to be pickier when shopping for clothing: Nothing with darts. Dark colors better than light. Some materials are better than others. Nothing low-cut. But, on the plus side, imagine this: no mammograms. No bras! No bouncing when you run up the stairs. Being able to sleep on your belly. There *ARE* benefits! (On a side note: I donated all my bras to "Free the Girls", a non-profit that supports women who survived sex trafficking by helping them start their own businesses selling bras and other lingerie.)

My only regret is not emphatically specifying I wanted to be *FLAT*. I believe my surgeon suspected I might change my mind about reconstruction and I don't think a lot of consideration was given to what I would look like if I didn't reconstruct. So I was left with "dog ears" – lumpy and bumpy and lopsided. I have met several "flat friends" through Facebook communities and blogging, and I'm a little jealous at the smoothness many of them possess. (Yes, many are proud to share photos! I haven't been that brave yet.) So if you ever have to make this decision, and you opt for the flat route, take photos of what you want to look like and have the discussion with your surgeon. (Be relentless and make them promise!)

໓

Drains

As I was doing my pre-surgery homework (i.e., perusing the Internet), I was on a site looking at wigs and prosthetics and whatnot. I stumbled upon a product that intrigued me: a camisole that velcro'd in the front and that had 4 pockets. Pockets? Whatever for?

It turns out that, when you have a mastectomy (I suppose *any* surgery where you are removing something), you end up with drains. Lovely little tubes that come out under your armpits and / or breast area. These drains help remove fluid buildup in little pockets called seromas post-surgery. This was another thing that wasn't really explained to me ahead of time, so when I saw the product, I was a bit shocked! After all, if my breasts and tumor were removed, where would fluid actually accumulate? It turns out that any time tissue is damaged, your body produces a healing fluid to help the repair process.

I've heard of women who have their drains in for weeks on end, but I was fortunate that mine were removed after only two days and before I left the hospital. I guess I didn't really need to spend money on the camisole, but who knew? I did continue to have

26

some minor fluid buildup, but it was aspirated by needle at the surgeon's office at my weekly post-op appointments. In case you are wondering, the needle aspiration didn't hurt at all. Whew!

𝄞

Healing

I was surprised at how little pain I had and how quickly I healed. Bandages were wrapped around my chest for a few days, including an ace bandage for compression, but I didn't even require any narcotics. I was able to manage my pain with Motrin and ice packs. I acknowledge that this isn't necessarily everyone's experience, so I was grateful.

I was able to shower (YEA!) without restriction. I had read about women who were relegated to sponge baths during their post-op healing, but my bandages were covered with waterproof dressing so I was set. The waterproof bandages came off after a few days, as the body itself had formed it's own waterproof seal. Amazing.

I had some bruising, tenderness, and swelling, but the ice packs continued to be my best friends during this period. It was also helpful to hang out in my pajamas all day, since they were comfy and unrestrictive.

A few of my friends had taken me shopping before my surgery and they bought me several tops that buttoned in the front. These were helpful post-surgery, and post-PJs. I think they are even more beneficial for those who have reconstruction, so I'd recommend that (in addition to the PJs!).

Under and below my armpits felt numb after the surgery and, honestly, to this day, those areas are still a bit wonky. It's as if they were shot with Novocain that never wore off, and I guess it's not surprising that there was some collateral damage from the surgery. Interestingly enough, my armpit hair doesn't really grow any more. I'm not sure if that's from the surgery, chemotherapy, or just menopause, but I just thought that was weird. I'm not really complaining, but, yeah. More weird.

𝄞

Sentinel Node Biopsy

Nothing I read in advance of my surgery prepared me for the sentinel node biopsy process. This process helps your surgeon determine if your cancer has spread to any lymph nodes, if s/he determines this is necessary.

The "sentinel" nodes are the first few nodes into which your tumor drains. [32] Once they are identified, they are flagged so that the surgeon knows which node(s) to remove during your breast surgery. They want to retain as many nodes as possible, so they remove the sentinels and analyze them in a lab while you are still in surgery. Depending on the results of that analysis, they may decide to take additional nodes if they think the spread goes beyond those first few.

It seems there are a few ways the sentinel node biopsy is done, based on surgeon preference. I had the "radioactive solution" injected. Yes, it was as fun as that sounds. Basically, I had four injections around my nipple, near the tumor location, of what I will call radioactive bee stings. Imagine a bee sting on your nipple. Now imagine that bee is injecting something radioactive.

I know. You can't really imagine it, can you? It was truly *THE* most painful thing I have ever endured. Yes, more painful than childbirth. No, I was not numbed. No, there was not anesthesia. (I have read that general anesthesia is sometimes used and I'm hoping that's more of a trend now.)

Gratefully, the pain subsided, somewhat quickly – about 15-30 seconds after each shot. The technician gave me permission to scream (many women have), gave me the option to do them quickly or take a break in between shots (I opted for get-it-over-quick), and was super compassionate through the process. My only thought at the time, however sexist it may sound, was "If this procedure had to be done to a man, you can bet your ass they'd be knocked out first!"

Once the radioactive solution was injected, the technician periodically checked via imaging if the solution had been taken up by the lymph nodes. Once they "lit up", he marked the location so the surgeon knew which nodes to remove. The goal is to remove as few nodes as possible, to prevent the risk of lymphedema. The lymphatic system performs a very important function, so the goal is preserve as many as they can. The days of removing all the nodes are in the past.

I ended up with only two nodes removed. Whew. The initial pathology on the day of the surgery indicated there was no evidence of cancer metastasis. The nodes were sent out post-surgery for additional analysis that indicated there *was* a micro-metastasis in my nodes, which my surgeon called "garbage cells". It was believed that there was no further infiltration into other nodes.

I am extremely grateful that I had such limited lymph node invasion considering the large size of my tumor. I feel like I dodged a bullet on that.

I was only out of work for two weeks after my surgery. This was a bit disappointing, as I was looking forward to being a couch potato and was not in a hurry to get back to work. By comparison, I was out of work for six weeks when I had my kidney cancer surgery in 2008. When I whined to my surgeon, he explained that an *internal* surgery is more invasive to the body, with more healing involved (muscles cut and things like that). But a mastectomy is *external* with limited healing challenges. Keep in mind this would be very different for someone who opted for reconstruction. In reality, I was feeling great and had no problems returning to work.

☨

Lymphedema

Lymphedema sometimes occurs after damage to the lymphatic system, such as surgical removal of one or more lymph nodes. Your lymph nodes are rather important little buggers and it's always best to have as few removed as possible. The more you have removed, the greater your chance of having lymphedema, but it can occur with removal of just one.

What happens with lymphedema is swelling – usually in your arms or legs – near where the nodes were removed. So with breast cancer, it normally appears in your arms.

Someone explained lymph nodes as being the trash collectors of the body. So if you remove a few, your garbage may sit on the curb and start to build up over time. The flow of the garbage through the lymphatic system and out of the body is compromised and fluid builds up in your limbs. In some cases, this fluid buildup is quite severe and can be debilitating. This was another topic that I stumbled upon accidentally, reading about it on a fellow breast cancer survivor's blog. I asked the question of my oncologist at some point post-treatment, and she said I had nothing to worry about because I had only had two nodes removed.

This was actually not the case – and that blog post said it only took one. But she reassured me, so I just went about my business. Then, on a weekend getaway with friends, exactly one year from my mastectomy, I did a lot of driving. I had overused my arm on this long trip and the next day, I had my first experience with lymphedema, although I didn't know that's what it was at the time.

My lymphedema did not result in the swelling of my arm, but rather swelling below my armpit. It was tender and swollen. Because of the pain, discomfort, and limited mobility of my right arm, I also ended up with range of motion issues.

I spent several weeks in physical and occupational therapy to help with the range of motion and to address the lymphedema. I learned how to do lymphatic massage during that time and now I just do it myself when I have a flare up. I am lucky that my lymphedema is not severe and doesn't impact my arm. I usually only get a flare up when I over use my arm (too much or too heavy). As soon as I feel it coming on, I start the lymphatic massage a few times a day and it usually goes away in a few days. Many, however, are living with this day in and day out, impacting their normal functioning, and requiring the wearing of compression sleeves.

§

Overall, I fared pretty well after the surgery. Around this time, I started eating better, juicing fruits and veggies, and managing my stress better, because next up was the thing I feared most: chemotherapy.

CHAPTER 5

Treatment & Side Effects: Chemotherapy

*"Courage is not the absence of fear, but rather the judgment that
something else is more important than one's fear."*
~ Ambrose Redmoon [33]

On August 2, 1996, I watched my first husband get infused with
his first chemo drug. He had been diagnosed with acute
lymphoblastic leukemia just one week prior and there he was:
starting chemo before we could barely comprehend what was
happening. I remember this day like it happened yesterday.

Ray was in an isolation room – not because he needed to be, but
because it was the only bed available on the very busy oncology
floor. The nurse infusing the drug was in training and was being
watched closely by another supervising nurse. I remember quite
vividly this large, clear syringe with a bright red liquid in it. If we
didn't know any better, it could have passed for Kool-Aid. As she
injected the needle into his port, a drop of this "red death" (a well-
earned nickname for Adriamycin) fell onto his bed sheet. The
supervising nurse expressed some concern, while Ray brushed it
off with a "Don't worry about it." We were then advised that if
the "red devil" (another apropos moniker) touched his skin, it
could burn his skin. Now, I don't know if that was 100 percent
true, or if it would just cause an irritation of some kind, but it
scared the bejesus out of us both. If contact could burn your skin,
what the hell were we doing injecting it *inside his body?!* We
looked at each other, frightened, as the "push" continued.

Watching Ray go through chemotherapy off and on for 918 days
was hell. I saw all the things we fear when we hear the word
"chemotherapy": nausea, vomiting, diarrhea, hair loss, bloating
from steroids, loss of energy, fatigue, and loss of quality of life.

31

Leukemia was a nasty disease that eventually robbed Ray of his life, despite all the hell he went through.

Flash forward 13+ years and now it was my turn. Those memories haunted me and I was terrified.

ঽ

I was back to work one whole day before I needed a day off to have my portacath surgically inserted. (I later had surgery for removal of the port several weeks after I finished radiation.) This would be the device through which I would receive my chemo, eliminating the need for the nurse to start a new line for each treatment. I was expecting a port similar to Ray's, which had two external "tails" through which blood was drawn and drugs were given where, once inserted, no additional needle pricks were ever needed.

My portacath was the kind that goes under the skin, so even when I received chemo, it still required a needle to be inserted through my skin. I'm sure there were other advantages, but since I still had to get stuck, I wondered what the point of it was. In fact, when I went for my blood work in between treatments, I would just request a regular vein draw just because it was easier and less painful.

I likened the needle to a pushpin on a cork bulletin board. When we first started using it, it actually hurt, as the skin was still tender from the surgical implant procedure. The nurses tried to numb it with this freezing spray, but that hurt too and didn't help much, so I opted to go without it after that first time.

In addition to the portacath, I had to get a MUGA Scan before starting chemo. This test baselines how well your heart functions. Basically, a MUGA measures the amount of blood pumped out of your heart with each heartbeat. A baseline is needed because some of the chemo can damage your muscles – including your heart. (Gulp.) Typically, a second MUGA is done at the conclusion of chemotherapy to see if there was any damage. I actually opted not to have the second one done because of the additional radiation. I figured as long as I was symptom free, I would take my chances. I had no prior history of heart issues, so my doctor accepted this choice.

X

My chemotherapy started on September 26, 2012. In order to make it as "fun" as humanly possible, my BFF, Leann, joined me. (If you ever have to go through this, I strongly recommend you get a Leann. Everyone needs one to make chemo – and life – bearable!)

The day got off to a rough start; we had arrived at 11:15 am but didn't see the oncologist until 1:15 pm. I was miffed at having to wait so long on what was an understandably stressful day. Luckily, I had my Leann and we were able to at least laugh while we waited and throughout the day.

I was blessed to have a fabulous oncology nurse who explained everything to me, in the detail that I wanted, answering all my questions from the drug info sheets. My day continued something like this:

- 2:00 pm – Emend drip (anti-nausea)
- 2:35 pm – Aloxi push (anti-nausea)
- 2:36 pm – Decadron drip (steroid)
- 3:00 pm – Taxotere (chemo)
- 4:15 pm – Adriamycin (chemo)
- 4:30 pm – Cytoxan (chemo)
- 5:15 pm – On my way home

A lovely six-hour day!

I highly recommend taking books, gaming devices, and movies - whatever you might enjoy to help kill some time. You might want to also take some comforts of home – your own pillow and blankey, for example, along with snacks. (Six hours is a long time!)

X

"AC-T" is a common breast cancer chemo combo.

Adriamycin is the very same drug that I watched Ray received all those years ago. I never imaged I'd be having the same thing done to me. My nurse said, "She's a good girl and does good things, but she has a nasty side." (Hey, sign me up!)

Cytoxan - don't you just love a drug with "tox" in the name? Oh, yes, give me some toxins.

Taxotere required the nurse to sit by my side for 15 minutes to make sure I didn't have a reaction. Scary. I never asked but was curious what kind of reactions were possible and what would they do. My big learning from the info sheet was that Taxotere was made from the Pacific Yew Tree. (I really did read everything!)

I was scheduled to receive six AC-T treatments, every three weeks.

On the way home, I grabbed my anti-nausea drugs from the pharmacy (Compazine and Zofran), which I (thankfully) rarely used.

Then the waiting game ensued. How long until I feel like crap? How bad will I feel? How soon until I lose my hair? Will I be able to work? Just how sick will I get?

℟

Day Two lulled me into a false sense of security. With steroids still flowing through my system, I felt pretty darn good. I went to the oncology office to get my Neulasta shot, which helped boost my white cells while chemo was damaging them. An equal opportunity destroyer, chemo takes the good along with the bad cells.

A side effect of Neulasta is bone pain, which I did deal with frequently. The recommendation was Tylenol and Claritin to manage the pain. They aren't really sure why Claritin helps, since that's not its original purpose, but it did work, so yea!

It is recommended that you drink a lot of water while on chemo and I am a notoriously bad water drinker. The recommendation was 64-96 ounces per day. I did my best.

I was always able to work on Day Two (the power of steroids), but by Day Three - Bam! I was down for the count. I would then generally sleep for 2½ days, waking up every few hours to eat, drink and pee. I'd then go back to work until the next chemo.

Lather. Rinse. Repeat.

ϰ

Side Effects

I know that I made it through chemo relatively unscathed compared to most people. I think it helped that I was eating healthier, taking a probiotic to help with nausea and diarrhea, juicing, sleeping when tired, and focusing on self-care. Not everyone has the luxury to do all that and everyone responds differently, and/or may be receiving different medications.

Following is a description of all of the side effects I endured, in no particular order. Some are short term, occurring while undergoing chemotherapy; others are longer term, happening well after I finished. Many of the short-term side effects are commonly known, but those long-term effects – they caught me completely off guard.

ϰ

Hair Loss

Having had fine, thin hair my entire life, losing my hair was an expectation. I think what threw me was just how quickly it happened. It took exactly 14 days. It came out in clumps, and I think I shed more than our German Shepherd. For not having much hair to start with, it did seem to get all over the place.

I had ordered a wig from a local business that supports women with breast cancer. The wig selection process was not as simple as you might imagine. Given my hair texture, I found most wigs to actually have too much hair. They didn't look like my hair at all. We kept trying and finally found something that worked. I highly recommend taking a few friends with you who will be honest with their opinions.

The cost of the wig was $300 and it was not covered by insurance. I wish I had known how little I would wear it, because I would have saved the money. I wore it about a week before tossing it in the closet. I found it to be hot and itchy, and I spent too much time worrying about if it was on straight. I was always tugging at it and looking in mirrors. As soon as I got in the car after work, I would immediately rip it off my head. Ultimately, I invested in scarves and wore those every day. Light, comfortable and fashionable, the scarves I wore were pre-tied with a bit of elastic in the back to hold them on. I have been able to share my collection of scarves with several other women undergoing chemotherapy, so we have definitely gotten our money's worth out of them. Interestingly, no one else has been interested in the wig either, so think carefully before spending your money on this.

I had heard many stories of people whose hair came in "different" post-chemo. I was hoping and praying for some thickness, maybe a bit of curl. Hey, why not a redhead? Alas, my hair came in pretty much the same, only thinner and finer. That wasn't really the "different" I was hoping for! It took about three months before anything noticeable showed up on my head and I felt comfortable going *sans scarf*. But at least I have hair, for which I am grateful, and I'll never have another bad hair day. Perspective.

In terms of hair in other places, my eyebrows mostly fell out and sort of came back, although somewhat sparse. They appear to grow places they shouldn't these days. I hate to pluck any, given they are few in numbers, but I do find myself plucking some and penciling in others. My eyelashes were never spectacular to begin with and are less so now. Mascara is our friend. I already mentioned the lack of hair under my pits, but I'm not really missing that at all. My leg hair is mostly back to normal although I don't think I shave nearly as much as I used to pre-chemo. Chin hair? Ugh, why are *those* the hairs that came back in force?

ʟ

Compromised Immune System

Two weeks for hair loss, but it took even less time for my immune system to be destroyed. Six whole days! When I returned to the oncologist after my first chemo treatment, I was advised that my white blood cell count was "nothing point nothing". In actuality, it was 1.8 (low end of normal is 4.0) but I believe the physician's assistant was trying to make a point. After swearing off antibiotics after the septic incident, I knew I'd have to give in here. Antibiotics can be your friend when used appropriately, and this was certainly one of those times.

In general, there were a lot of ebbs and flows with my immune system, as was expected. The healthy cells are killed off with the cancer cells when you receive chemo, so your counts dip and then come back gradually.

The best bet is to sit your butt home during those ebbs, and to avoid contact with sick people. My staff and friends at work were great about calling me to say, "Everyone here is hacking! Stay home!" Again, I was fortunate to have the opportunity to work from home when needed; I know most people are not so lucky and will be required to take sick time.

Food and the Gastro-Intestinal System

As much as I was trying to eat healthier during this time, I found my taste buds were some of the first casualties of chemo. Food started to taste funny; it was often very metallic tasting, and many textures grossed me out. Despite trying to limit sugar (does sugar really feed cancer?), I was actually drawn to sugary foods. It was the only taste that remained true to form. Sugar still tasted like sugar. But all those healthy, plant-based foods I was trying to consume? Not so much.

I did the best I could. I ate healthy when I could tolerate the tastes, and I ate sweets when my buds rejected everything else. My go-to treat was my mom's homemade rice pudding – eggs, milk and sugar –all the things I was trying to avoid. However, at some point, you just need the calories. I'm sure there were some healthier things I could have eaten that would have worked, but since others were helping to cook for me, I just went with it.

When I decided to go 100 percent plant based post-chemo, the crazy-taste-buds thing helped me a lot. All I had to do was remember the texture of hamburger in my mouth, and - ew!

In terms of nausea, I made out pretty well: minor nausea in the beginning and only vomiting a few times after round six because of chemo's cumulative effects. I did take a probiotic every day and, while I'm not sure if that's exactly what did the trick, it certainly didn't hurt. Other contributing factors, perhaps: juicing fruits and vegetables and eating high fiber foods whenever possible. These actions also benefited me in the bathroom as well. And we'll leave it there, lest we tread into Too Much Information.

Fatigue / Insomnia / Restless Legs

As mentioned earlier in this chapter, I slept a lot immediately following chemo. The fatigue from the treatments didn't surprise me or bother me too much, but the insomnia that followed the first few sleep-filled days was just as exhausting. I had trouble falling asleep *AND* staying asleep because of restless legs. It was believed the leg issue was due to the Neulasta shots. Claritin was recommended and it did help a bit, but still, sleep was often elusive.

※

Hiccups

While this may seem like a pretty tame side effect, it can be a real annoyance. I frequently had the hiccups, which were likely the cause of nerve irritation, the chemo drugs, and/or problems in the brain [34], which leads me to…

※

Chemo Brain

I had heard about chemo brain (more formally known as "chemotherapy-related cognitive impairment") and I can attest to its existence. While not definitively linked to the chemo itself, the drugs do tend to get the blame (personally, I was fine before the drugs, so I'm inclined to blame drugs myself). With chemo brain, there may be problems with memory, concentration, or language. [35] The struggle is real. I dealt with forgetfulness at a whole new level, and struggle even to this day. This goes beyond forgetting why you went to the fridge, or why you entered a room. It's embarrassing to forget the name of someone you've known your whole life. I do miss those brain cells!

※

Hearing Loss

I have to admit that this one surprised me. In 2015 I started having issues with my left ear. It felt like it was blocked all the time. I chalked it up to an ear infection or something like that, but it just wouldn't go away. It was worse if there was background noise, and I often had incessant ringing in my ear. After about six months or so, I decided to see a specialist for a hearing test. While I had some minor loss in my right ear, I had significant hearing loss in my left ear. I didn't realize that hearing loss feels like a blocked ear, or like you have water in it. At any rate, they had me go for an MRI to make sure there wasn't a tumor or something pressing on the nerves (and, thankfully, there was no tumor!), but the ENT did confirm that the hearing loss was related to nerve damage.

Learning that made me start thinking – many chemo patients get neuropathy, a nerve disorder that can cause numbness, among other things. I wondered if the hearing loss was possibly related to my chemotherapy. I ran to my computer as soon as I got home from the doctor's office and, sure enough, there it was on the list of long-term side effects. It doesn't always show up right away; in my case, it was two years later.

I am grateful, as a musician, that the loss is only in one ear, and I hope it stays that way. I do wear a hearing aid, which I don't even think about most days.

⚸

There are many more possible side effects, including secondary cancers, so (as always) I recommend doing your homework and asking a lot of questions.

As you can see, I did manage through better than most. While not pleasant in the least, I am fully aware it could have been worse – in many ways. I thought that chemo was the end of my treatment road, as that was what was communicated to me early on. But, as I neared the end of my chemotherapy regiment, my oncologist spoke of my referral to a radiation oncologist. I recall not being too pleased about that and was angry about being misled, but I kept my appointment, leading me to the next phase of my treatment.

CHAPTER 6

Treatment & Side Effects: Radiation

*"Radiation, unlike smoking, drinking, and overeating, gives no pleasure,
so the possible victims object."* ~ Isaac Asimov [36]

I was dead set against having radiation. I don't know why,
exactly, but I fought it. Perhaps it was because the expectation had
been set earlier that I didn't need it. Maybe it was the thought of
more radiation, after years of CT scans for my kidneys. I had
thoughts of Spiderman, the Incredible Hulk, and the movie,
Silkwood! (Dramatic, yes, but truthful.)

I really just wanted to be done with treatment and move on, so I
was pretty pissed when my oncologist brought it up. Since my
doctor recommended it, my husband encouraged me to proceed
with this part of the treatment, but I put the onus on the
radiologist to make his case.

My radiation oncologist presented a pretty compelling case to me.
I believe my oncologist gave him the head's up that I was going to
be a tough nut to crack, and he was prepared – with charts and
graphs and websites and DVDs and pamphlets. He demonstrated
that protocol, based on my exact tumor size/type/lymph
invasion, warranted radiation. He explained that chemotherapy is
your insurance policy against metastasis, and radiation is your
insurance policy against rogue cells that might remain at the
cancer site. This is particularly important when you tumor is eight
centimeters. He was also a pretty persuasive speaker, so, in the
end, he got me to agree. By the time the radiation phase was all
over, he had become a trusted advisor to me.

ጸ

Before radiation actually starts, there are some preparatory actions. First was the creation of a custom mold of my head and arms over my head that would ensure my body was in the exact same position every time I went for radiation.

Second was getting tattooed; these small marks help the technicians line up the machines each time. It's all about precision. I like to tell people I have three tattoos, and it isn't a lie, but they are about the size of dot you make when you drop your ink pen! One was placed in the middle of my sternum, and then one on either side under my armpits. For the record, despite my getting sick of getting stuck with needles, the tattoos didn't hurt at all.

The day prior to actually starting radiation, I went for a dry run for purposes of calibrating machines, paperwork, and a walk through of the process. I was scheduled for 35 total radiation treatments, which included seven "boosters" on my mastectomy scar.

On the day of my first treatment, I changed into my hospital gown (top only) and readied myself for this weird experience. When called, I was walked back into the room where the dry run occurred – a room with an enormously thick door that protected the technicians from excessive exposure. It occurred to me that waiting for that door to open and close each time would drive me crazy (not being a patient person of any kind). I lay down on the metal table and was positioned in my mold. You aren't allowed to move and the technicians move your body parts around to get you into the EXACT position.

The technician is obviously not in the room during the actual treatment, but you can see them in the window (sort of – remember, you can't move). The machines rotate around you and there is some strange buzzing. I now know what it feels like to be a baked potato in the microwave! The process never took more than 10 minutes or so, and then I was on my way. For me, treatments were scheduled after work, so I could head out on time, get my radiation, and go home.

ঙ

As someone who believes in natural remedies, I took the advice of my fabulous naturalist and took a 20-minute Epsom salt and baking soda bath every day after radiation. This was to protect my thyroid, by helping to remove the radiation from my body. (I also took an iodine supplement during this time.) Whether you believe in such things or not, I still recommend this practice as a means of stress relief and self-care. Just add three cups of Epsom salts plus one cup of baking soda to a hot bath; soak for 20 minutes only.

ஃ

I'm almost embarrassed to say, similarly to chemotherapy, I feel like I skated through radiation relatively unscathed. I know I shouldn't feel badly about not feeling bad, but so many others have had it so much worse that I do feel a bit of guilt. I do know how bad it can be and how lucky I was.

I did not experience any fatigue, and I had no issues with skin irritation, burning, or blistering. I wish the same could have been said for many of the women I met in the waiting room. There were a number of women I met who really struggled with the burning and blistering. Clothing (especially bra straps) further irritated the site. These women were often in tears and struggled to continue therapy. My heart broke seeing them in such pain.

The most common side effects of radiation include fatigue and skin issues, and effects can vary greatly from person to person, depending on the exact location of the treatment. Radiation is done at the site of the tumor only, but, for example, if you had radiation to the head, you could have hair loss. Radiation to the abdomen could result in nausea. My dad, who had parotid gland cancer, had radiation to head/neck area and suffered from a great deal of fatigue. There are a number of more severe side effects, including a rare situation of a secondary cancer (it always scared me a little that most of my treatments could cause the very thing I was trying to beat). I won't be covering them all here, but if you should ever need radiation, what should you do?

You know it: Do your homework and ask lots of questions.

I think it bears mentioning that there is a limit to the amount of radiation you can receive in your lifetime. Depending on how much radiation you need for treatment, it is possible that you wouldn't be able to receive radiation a second time. [37] This is yet another reason to focus on self-care and reducing your risks.

Onward to the final step.

CHAPTER 7

Treatment & Side Effects: Hormone Therapy

"Hormones get no respect. We think of them as the elusive chemicals that make us a bit moody, but the magical molecules do so much more."
~Susannah Cahalan [38]

When you have a hormone receptive tumor, the last step in the treatment process is hormone therapy. Since the tumor benefited from the presence of the estrogen and progesterone, this part of your treatment helps to reduce the amount of hormones in your body, which would slow or halt any additional growth. I was advised that ER and PR positive breast cancers are easier to treat and have the most success due to this additional piece of treatment.

☣

For pre-menopausal women, Tamoxifen is usually the drug of choice and is the most commonly known. It is usually taken for 5-10 years and works by stopping estrogen from attaching to any cancer cells to prevent them from growing. There are a number of possible side effects from this drug, including hot flashes, fatigue, headache, mood swings, and more. [39]

As someone who was menopausal, I was placed on an aromatase inhibitor (AI). These drugs stop estrogen production, which in turn starves any cancer cells. There are three commonly used AIs: Arimidex, Aromasin and Femara. Initially, I was advised I would be going on Aromasin, but that was changed to Femara. (Note: There are other drugs for metastatic breast cancer that will not be covered here.)

With some hesitation, since I was trying to avoid all unnatural chemicals in my body, I started taking the Femara a few weeks

43

after my radiation ended. AIs also have a slew of side effects, but the ones to really impact me were night sweats and insomnia. While I didn't experience a lot of menopausal symptoms before, I was certainly experiencing them on this drug. Sleep went something like this: Too hot. Uncover. Too cold. Cover. Toss. Turn. Hot again. This all resulted in night after night of sleeplessness. And all I could think was: *I have to do this for five years?!?!*

After a few weeks of not sleeping, the joint pain started. Particularly in my knees and feet, the pain also spread to my hips, shoulders, and hands. I had trouble moving, and getting out of bed in the morning was the worse. I felt about 100 years old and the pain often brought tears to my eyes. I took glucosamine and curcumin, swallowed Tylenol like candy, and even added gobs of ginger root to my juices to help with inflammation and pain – all with limited success.

About six weeks in, I was at my wit's end. I wanted to quit this medication but was afraid of a recurrence. So what's worse: intolerable pain for five years and no quality of life, or fear of cancer's return? I continued with it but managed to frequently "forget" to take it. I even gave myself a weeklong vacation from the drug at one point.

At three months, I broached the subject with my oncologist. The answer was to prescribe additional drugs for the side effects. Not sleeping? You can take a sleeping pill. Pain? Try Motrin. (As if I had not already tried that...) Hot flashes? Try Vitamin E. (Really?) Elevated blood pressure? Well, of course, you can have a blood pressure pill.

My oncologist felt like there were "no options" for me except to continue on the Femara. I had other thoughts on my options: How about not taking it? Good, bad or indifferent, it's still an option. Or how about trying one of the others? I walked away from the conversation frustrated but determined to do my own research on my options. And research I did.

In the meantime, I stopped taking it to manage my side effects. After three months of not sleeping, I was ready to snap. This decision was not taken lightly. I felt guilty for not taking it, especially because I hadn't confessed to anyone initially. I continued to be afraid of a recurrence and felt I should "do everything," but how could I keep living like this? So I'd take it for a few days, then stop again. That wasn't the best option either.

§

I started my research by trying to learn all about the importance of hormones. I mean they *do* serve a purpose, right? We tend to associate hormones with reproductive functions, but they do so much more than that. As the quote at the beginning of this chapter states, they *are* magical molecules. Powerful little messengers that control most major bodily functions. [40] Yeah, that's right: Most. Major. Functions.

Insufficient hormone levels can contribute to many diseases: diabetes, high blood pressure, fatigue, thyroid disease, and more. Low estrogen, specifically, can result in hot flashes, osteoporosis, painful intercourse, and weight gain, to name a few.

Vaginal atrophy is actually a thing; it is a thinning, drying and inflammation of the vaginal walls – and I got it. Ditto on the lichen sclerosus, with which I was also diagnosed. Both resulted in the terribly painful intercourse for me and I needed to find ways to fix this.

I had Femara, menopause, and fried ovaries going against me.

§

In addition to reading everything I could get my hands on and surfing the Internet, I decided to take advantage of an employee benefit offered by my employer: Best Doctors. This service allowed me to get a second opinion from an expert in the field of medicine associated with my diagnosis. I could not recommend this service more! It was a wealth of information for me through their "Ask the Expert" services. In addition to having them review *ALL* my medical records to confirm diagnosis and treatment plan, I got to spend an hour on the phone with an expert, asking all the questions that I struggled to get answers to.

What I really wanted to know was: If I already did surgery, chemotherapy and radiation, what was my risk if I stopped the Femara? What was my prognosis, with and without the AI?

I learned that my estimated 10-year survival rate was 77 percent with the use of chemo and hormone therapy (it didn't seem to account for the radiation therapy, and was slightly lower than other estimates as a result). The 77 percent was related to death by any reason, not necessarily just breast cancer. Not taking the Femara would reduce my survival rate by roughly 5 percent. In weighing the loss of quality of life, which was pretty poor on this drug, against the loss of 5 percent on my survival rate, I opted for the latter.

Armed with this information, I returned to my oncologist, presented the data to her, and got her approval to stop taking it.

Please know that I am NOT recommending this for everyone. For me, it was the right decision. I was dealing with horrible pain and no sleep, day after day, month after month (for six months). I had regular headaches, UTI-type symptoms (without presence of a UTI), shooting pain down my arms, and more. I couldn't function. I couldn't figure out what was a side effect and what was a real symptom of something to be concerned with. It was the right decision for me.

During this time, I was also making a number of significant lifestyle changes – improved nutrition being the most significant – and I felt those changes helped to mitigate any future risks. Before I talked to my oncologist, I also sought counsel from my radiologist and gynecologist, both of whom supported my decision.

As with every other discussion point in this book, do talk to your doctor. Ask questions. Use every resource you can to make informed decisions that are the best for YOU. Only you can decide, but you have to be armed with data.

ॐ

With the Femara now gone, I was able to set my sights on feeling better. It took months before the joint pain and insomnia really went away, but I felt better just having the weight of that decision off my shoulders. With my gynecologist's help, I managed to heal the lichen sclerosus and vaginal atrophy with supplementation and Estriol.

Estriol is the weakest of the three principal estrogens: estrone, estradiol, and estriol. [41] Because of its lower potency, many doctors believe it can help manage hormone-related symptoms (such as those described above) without the dangers related to estrogen-positive cancer. In order to try this particular hormone for my issues, my gynecologist and I did a lot of research before agreeing to give it a shot. We both felt it would provide benefits while not risking a recurrence. I now use it vaginally only twice a week, and it has alleviated both the lichen sclerosus and the vaginal atrophy, along with other menopausal symptoms. [42] It does require a prescription and is not widely available. I obtain my estriol cream from a compounding pharmacy in a nearby town. There is still a lot of debate on the use of estriol, but it has worked for me and I have had no negative effects from it. It may not be appropriate for everyone, but I thought it was worth discussing here.

In addition to the estriol, I also help manage my hormone issues using supplements. You can read more about that in Chapter 11.

⚲

After all my treatments, I was ready to leave all the cancer stuff behind me to focus on the future. Unfortunately, cancer never really leaves you. Years out, I still worry about a recurrence – not as often as in the early years, but it always lingers in the back of my brain. Every illness or symptom wakens that fear. In a way, that fear is what keeps me from getting too complacent on my self-care, so I suppose it serves a useful purpose. I think it's important to not let it consume you too much and just focus on what you can control, like diet!

CHAPTER 8

Healing Your Body: The Power of Nutrition

*"The food you put into your body is the single most powerful
factor that determines your health and well-being."*
~ John McDougall, MD [43]

Did you know that:

- As many as 40 percent of cancers are due to poor diet? [44]

- There are some foods that have been deemed
  carcinogenic? Meaning they can actually *cause* cancer? [45]

- Whole Food Plant Based Diets have been proven to reverse
  disease? Yes, you read that right: reverse! They can help
  prevent disease, as well. (Check out the list of resources in
  Chapter 14 to learn more about this.)

In my experience, no one ever really talks about the impact of diet
on our health; surprisingly, it's been rare for me even in the
medical community. Sure, we all talk about "diet-ing", but the
focus is always on losing weight and *looking* good, and rarely on
nutrition and *feeling* good. Most diets, if followed with some level
of discipline, will result in weight loss – and simply losing weight
has a lot of great benefits in the short term. Yet, very few of them
are truly healthy in the long term, and even fewer talk about
actually *nourishing* your body. You know, feeding it nutrients to
optimize your health.

I spent years "diet-ing" – counting calories, counting points,
counting grams of fat and sugar – but I spent no time measuring
quality. I ate my share of frozen "healthy" meals. I used packaged

foods to help make dinner. I thought "low-fat" packaging meant it was good for me. In retrospect, I know now that it was all junk. Health is about so much more than calories in, calories out. The quality of those calories really matters. If you have 100 calories of potato chips and 100 calories of an apple, which do you think will yield the better health outcome?

In this chapter and the next, I will share some of what I have learned about nutrition and how it dramatically improved my health. I absolutely believe that a healthy diet can reverse disease and maybe even prevent us from getting disease in the first place. And isn't prevention better than a cure?

ℛ

At the time of my breast cancer diagnosis, I knew I needed to do something different. This was my second cancer diagnosis, and I believed, if I didn't make changes, I was going to die. My son was only 11 at the time, and I had to fight for the chance to see him grow up. I wasn't exactly sure where to start, but, oddly, I remembered reading in a magazine a few years prior about a cancer documentary with the words "crazy" and "sexy" in the title. I didn't remember the details, but those words were enough to get me started. In fact, it would be the catalyst to my health journey.

After Googling "crazy sexy cancer", I discovered Kris Carr's book, *Crazy Sexy Diet*. This was my first foray into nutrition-focused health books. It was funny, fascinating, and educational, and it led me to many more resources (see Chapter 14 for a full list of recommendations). I could not stop consuming everything I could find on the topic of plant-based nutrition – books, documentaries, blogs, cookbooks – and I became convinced that this was the answer for me. It was the book *The China Study* that really led me to understand the connection of animal protein with cancer. After reading that book, I realized that I had nothing to lose, and everything to gain.

ℛ

So how does a plant-based diet work to fight cancer, anyway?

- It boosts your immune system through phytonutrients.
- Cancer-fighting antioxidants are mainly found in vegetables and fruits.
- A plant-based diet is naturally anti-angiogenic, meaning it prevents the growth of blood vessels that feed tumors/cancer. [46]
- By eating foods that are less-calorie dense, you will feel fuller while consuming fewer calories, thus losing weight. Being a healthy weight, as we discussed, reduces your cancer risk.
- Diets high in fiber and low in fat tend to reduce estrogen in the body.
- Dairy products tend to increase insulin-like growth factor 1 (IGF-1) which has been linked to breast and ovarian cancer.
- Cooked meats generate cancer-causing heterocyclic amines that may cause cancer. [47]

ॐ

I started slow, focusing only on myself initially. Eventually I (mostly) transitioned my husband and son to this diet, as well. My son still eats meat at school and when he's away; my hubby is more a lacto-ovo-vegetarian since he doesn't want to give up cheese and eggs.

What is a lacto-ovo-vegetarian? I'm glad you asked.

I view eating habits on a continuum and often coach clients to look at where they are and try to move, even in small steps, along the spectrum towards improved nutrition. It looks something like this:

⇓ **Omnivores** – eat pretty much anything

⇓ **Pescatarians** – don't eat meat, but do eat fish

⇓ **Flexitarians** – eat mostly plant based, but occasionally indulge in meat/fish

⇓ **Vegetarians** – all plants, plus

⇓ **Lacto-Vegetarians** – consume dairy products

⇓ **Ovo-Vegetarians** – consume eggs

⇓ **Lacto-Ovo-Vegetarians** – yep, you got it! Both dairy and eggs

⇓ **Vegans**

> *Ethical Vegans* do not eat anything related to animals (this usually includes honey) and also do not wear animals (no leather, etc.). The term ethical vegan is used more to describe a philosophy than a diet and relates to humane treatment of animals, but certainly diet is part of it. Not all vegan diets are super healthy, as some may be consuming processed or fried foods. For example, Oreo cookies and French fries are vegan, but not necessarily the healthiest choices.

> *Plant Based* – refers to diets that derived solely from plants. There are variations within this category as well: Fruitarians and Raw Vegans, as examples.

> *Whole Food Plant Based No Oil* – To really up your game to the mother of all vegetarian/vegan diets, there is the WFPBNO diet. This is what I strive for every day, although I'm not perfect by any stretch of the imagination. This diet excludes meat, fish, eggs, dairy, and added oils.

⚡

I went 100 percent meat-free at the conclusion of my chemotherapy, but still ate some fish, cooked with oils, and ate cheese and eggs. It took a trip to California, several more books, and trial-and-error to reach WFPBNO.

The trip to California was to attend a weekend conference hosted by Dr. John McDougall. I had not yet discovered Dr. McDougall's work, but many of the rock stars of the plant-based world were speaking at this event and I knew I had to go. I was grateful to find a friend to go along for the ride and, off we went. If I had any doubts about this diet *before* I attended this conference, I was completely convinced at the end of our three days. The speakers were a wealth of information and I learned the importance of the "no oil". WFPBNO became a new religion, of sorts. After all, I had eaten a boatload of food over that conference weekend and managed to lose three pounds. They were certainly on to something!

ɤ

Even though I was not eating meat, it took me a while to actually stop cooking meat completely. I still had a family to feed, and I wasn't going to force this on them. For a long while, it was all about me. I bought a number of cookbooks and started experimenting. Whatever I made for myself became the side dish for my family – along with their chicken or fish or whatever.

Over time, I identified the dishes that my family enjoyed and, ever so gradually, I stopped cooking meat altogether. If this diet was good for *MY* health, then surely it would help my family as well. In fact, my son, an avid milk drinker, stopped drinking cow's milk after we were doing this a while. Do you know what else stopped? Six trips to the doctor every year for strep throat and ear infections. No lie. My husband, who ate Prilosec and Tums like they were candy, suddenly no longer required medication of any kind for acid reflux.

As for me, I dropped 20 pounds. My cholesterol dropped to the mid-100s (There is no cholesterol in plants! I had never thought about that before). My triglycerides fell over 100 points. My blood pressure was a cool 90/60. My skin became clearer and brighter, I had more energy than ever before, and I felt amazing.

All of this without giving up a bit of enjoyment! The foods we eat are delicious, simple, and diverse. Our weekly menu is far more interesting now than it ever was as omnivores. I experiment with spices I had never heard of before, and our meals are now more international – Italian, Greek, Lebanese, Asian, Indian, and plant-based versions of our favorite American foods.

ɤ

Six years out, I wish I could say my diet is still perfect, but it's not. I do occasionally indulge in some cheese or seafood, but it's rare. I don't stress about whether something I'm eating in a restaurant has a bit of oil or maybe an egg as an ingredient. I think you could drive yourself a little batty stressing over every morsel and it's important to find the right balance – and by balance, I do not mean 50/50. I mean 95/5 or 99/1. Shoot for "never" eating those foods, and if they slip in here and there, I think you'll be ok.

That said, I absolutely believe that anyone with a serious chronic illness would benefit greatly from the WFPBNO diet. It is the only diet that has ever been proven to prevent and reverse disease. I have seen the healing properties of this diet in my own life and in many of my clients who stuck to it faithfully. I believe if you are chronically ill, whether it's cancer, heart disease, diabetes, or whatever, you need to follow this diet 100 percent to see results. Doing it part-time will yield part-time results and you will never heal. The progress would be so slow as to be ineffective.

CHAPTER 9

Healing Your Body: How To Eat Right

"The food you eat can be either the safest and most powerful form of medicine, or the slowest form of poison." ~ Ann Wigmore [48]

Food as medicine really comes down to two pieces: Avoiding foods that make us sick, and consuming foods that nourish and heal. Easy, right? When we stop to think about it, deep down, we all know what foods are healthy and which are not. We know it. So why don't we do it?

We eat out of boredom or convenience. We eat when we're happy – and when we're sad. We connect food to families and traditions. We are *so* attached to our foods, but remember this:

Nothing tastes as good as healthy feels.

Nothing.

If it meant you could have your health back, wouldn't you want to at least try?

⚹

In order to avoid foods that make us sick and cause cancer, we need to be clear about what those foods are.

IARP (International Agency for Research on Cancer) puts out a list of foods that have been classified as Group 1 carcinogens, meaning they cause cancer in humans. One of the top items on the list: processed meats. That means hot dogs, deli meats, and the beloved bacon. [49, 50]

Sorry for all you bacon-lovers. (Ok, not sorry.)

To be blunt, it's no different than smoking cigarettes and then being surprised that you get lung cancer. These foods *cause cancer*. So just stop. If you really need your bacon fix, I can hook you up with a great mushroom bacon recipe that's to die for. (Pun intended.)

Other Group 1 carcinogens in our diets include alcohol (another tough one for many), Chinese-style salted fish (I'm not really sure what that is), burned or heavily barbecued foods, red meat and contaminated water. [50]

⚘

While not a Group 1 carcinogen, I do recommend staying away from added oils in your diet. When I say this to people, I usually get the deer-in-the-headlights look, followed by, "But I thought olive oil was good for me." Or, "Don't we need fats in our diet?" Or, "Impossible!"

This is certainly a topic of debate amongst many medical professionals, as well as many people who I know have healed themselves with food. I respect all of their opinions, and you can certainly do more research on your own, but I would like to share my rationale for no oil.

First, oil isn't a "whole food". Olives are a whole food; olive *oil* is a processed food.

Second, oils are 100 percent fat. No protein, no carbs. One tablespoon of olive oil contains 14 grams of fat and 120 calories. As Dr. McDougall would say, "The fat you eat is the fat you wear." [51] If you are trying to lose weight, I ask you to consider the amount of oil you use to prepare your foods. How much are you *really* using? (Do you actually measure or do you just pour?) Now add that up over a week of meals. The oil you are cooking with can really slow your weight loss efforts and, as we have already discussed, being at a healthy weight lowers your risk of cancer.

Next, many oils are inflammatory, and inflammation leads to chronic disease, including cancer.

Lastly, oils contribute to heart disease by lessening endothelial function in your arteries. I'm not going to cover any of that here, since this is a book on cancer, and the topic is a bit beyond my expertise, but you can check out multiple resources by Dr. Caldwell Esselstyn for the best explanation on oils and heart disease.

I am not going to lie to you and say I never, ever use olive oil. I do cook on a giant cast iron pan from time to time, and that needs a spritz of oil before cooking. But it's a *spritz* from a spray bottle, not a *pour*. All of my other sautéing is done with vegetable broth or water. If you need to use a bit of olive oil as you start to eat healthier, look to eliminate it over time, and ALWAYS measure. Do not just blindly pour your oil into a pan, because I have no doubt you are using more than a tablespoon if you do.

𝓧

Now that you know what NOT to eat, let's talk about what you should eat. Does anyone want to take a guess? Yes, as we've all been told growing up: "Eat your fruits and vegetables!"

See? I told you we all know what's healthy!

Plants have all the nutrients we need (minus just a few which we'll cover in the chapter on supplementation):

- **Carbohydrates** – Carbs always seem to get a bum rap, especially with so much focus lately on low-carb diets. Whenever someone tells me they are cutting out carbs, I always ask them to be more specific. If, by carbs, you mean cookies and pastries and over-processed white bread, that's fine. But if you mean *all* carbs, that's when I'm going to express some concern. Carbohydrates are your body's main fuel source. Yes, carbs get broken down into glucose, but that's what is supposed to happen to fuel the cells in your brain, organs, and everywhere! Fruits, vegetables, whole grains, beans and legumes are all healthy sources of carbohydrates.

- **Protein** – Ask any vegetarian their most dreaded question and the answer will undoubtedly be "where do you get your protein?" To which we usually have a witty retort like "I get my protein where your protein gets its protein!" It may be surprising to know that plants do, indeed, have more than enough protein. The top sources of plant protein: tofu, lentils, beans, quinoa, seeds, nuts and nut butters. You may also be interested to know that you don't need as much protein as you think you do. The average woman only needs about 50 grams a day, and most of us are getting far more than that. [52] Too much protein can result in weight gain, constipation, heart disease, kidney damage, and increased cancer risk. [53]

- **Fiber** – Did you know that meat contains zero fiber? It's pretty much why everyone in the US is always so constipated! Fiber helps regulate bowel movements, lowers cholesterol levels, helps control blood sugar levels, and helps you maintain a healthy weight. Without sufficient fiber in your diet, your risk of colon cancer increases, and you are at higher risk of heart disease. Fiber rich foods include fruits, vegetables, lentils, beans, quinoa, and oats.

- **Vitamins and Minerals** – Fruits and veggies are chock full of the vitamins and minerals needed for good health, including, Vitamins A, C, and E, magnesium, potassium, zinc, folic acid, calcium, iron, and so much more. It's important to eat a variety of foods to ensure that you are getting a variety of vitamins and minerals. As they say, "Eat the rainbow"; the more color, the more nutrients.

- **Fats** – We discussed that WFPBNO means I do not cook with any added oils, but getting healthy fat into your diet is very important, in particular for the health of your brain and organs. Healthy, whole-food, plant-based sources of fat include avocados, nuts and nut butters, seeds, olives, and soy/tofu.

- **Omega-3 Fatty Acids** – These are important for brain health. In a plant-based diet, they are found in chia seeds, flax and walnuts. It's super easy to sprinkle these into a salad, soup, oatmeal, or other dish.

- **Water** – If you are a bad water drinker, like myself, consuming fruits and vegetables is a great way to help with hydration. Some fruits and veggies with high water content include *water*melon (of course!), strawberries, pineapple, oranges, cucumbers, and celery.

In addition to these essential nutrients, plants have the highest amount of antioxidants. These compounds fight against the free radicals that cause damage to your cells and DNA and are linked to several diseases, including cancer. Examples of foods rich in antioxidants include berries, beans, apples, potatoes, dark leafy greens, and onions/garlic. [54]

☙

What about soy? Avoiding soy was an explicit directive from my oncologist, since soy is a phytoestrogen, or plant estrogen, and I had an estrogen-positive tumor. So I avoided it for years (I didn't know what to do with it anyway), but I kept encountering articles that discussed the many benefits of soy. So which was it? Good or bad? I wasn't sure, so, when in doubt, don't.

That was until I read *How Not to Die* by Dr. Michael Greger. In his book, Dr. Greger details, with science behind him, all of the benefits of soy – including benefits for breast cancer. [55] I urge you to check out his videos on *nutritionfacts.org* related to soy and breast cancer for a very detailed explanation. [56] I can't really do it justice, but it involves how your body processes phytoestrogens. As a result of Dr. Greger's science-based explanations, I do now include tofu and tempeh in our weekly menu (and now I'm an expert tofu cooker!).

An important point when talking about soy is to differentiate between healthy sources of soy (tofu, edamame, tempeh, soy sauce, miso, soy milk) and UN-healthy sources (soy protein isolate, as an example, and all crappy processed soy in crappy processed foods). Be sure to purchase organic, non-GMO soy, if you decide to give it a try.

☙

There are so many sources of conflicting information on what constitutes a healthy diet, and we're all very different, so here are my recommendations for getting started:

1. **Incorporate cancer-fighting foods into your diet each day**
   Eat foods such as: berries, leafy greens, cruciferous vegetables like broccoli, kale, and cabbage (remember the Indole-3-Carbinol?), garlic, beans, mushrooms, and onions. Spice your meals up with the top cancer-fighting spices: oregano, garlic, cayenne, and turmeric.

2. **Be mindful of what you are eating**
   With every bite of food that you eat, be mindful of whether you are consuming healing foods, or if you are doing damage to your body. With that awareness of what you are eating, you are more likely to make healthier choices. This is especially important if you are already sick.

3. **Plan, plan, plan**
   Without a game plan, you are setting yourself up for failure. Take the time each week to sit down and thoughtfully plan your meals for the week. Think about your schedule: which nights might need a quick meal, when do you have to work late, what are the kids' schedules like, etc.? And then plan accordingly. Don't plan a meal with lots of chopping on a busy night.

   Have a Plan B for when Plan A goes awry, because it will. I always keep a few "quick meals" on hand – like whole-wheat pasta and jarred marinara sauce, or rice and beans.

   Use your menu plan to populate your grocery list. That will help ensure you are only buying what you need and nothing you don't. No wandering around the store trying to figure it out.

4. **Cook your own food**
   Restaurant foods are loaded with salt and fat; processed foods contain that and often a bunch of unrecognizable ingredients. Cooking your own food gives you total control over what does or does not go into the dish.

5. **Crowd out unhealthy foods**
   Before you even start eliminating certain foods, you can simply start adding healthy foods to crowd out the less healthy choices. For example, eat your veggies and starches first and you will end up eating less meat/fish, even if it's on your plate.

6. **Try something new**
   Variety is the spice of life! Try some new fruits or veggies, or a new grain or spice. Herbs and spices help keep your meals interesting and they provide an additional layer of nutrition. Packing a host of healing properties, some of the most powerful herbs and spices are: turmeric, ginger, cinnamon, parsley, cayenne, and cumin.

7. **Put your meals on autopilot**
   When starting out with a healthier diet, I found that it is easier to put at least a few meals on autopilot. What that means is: pick one option and eat it every day. For example, if you decide to eat oatmeal for breakfast, eat that every day. Do the same for lunch; same thing every day. Then you can mix up dinner, trying different foods and recipes. The benefit of autopilot is that you will not be so overwhelmed trying to plan 21 unique meals each week. As time goes on, you can vary what you eat for breakfast and lunch, as well.

I think it bears repeating that if you are already sick, you need to clean up your diet and go hard-core if you have any chance of healing your body. Our bodies are amazing machines that know how to fight disease, but we have to give them the proper fuel. We have to repair our gut health and strengthen our immune systems, and you simply can't do that on a junky diet.

I often hear from people that "disease runs in my family" – and I'm not totally dismissing genetics – but do you know what else runs in families? Unhealthy diets and lifestyle choices.

CHAPTER 10

Healing Your Body: Juices and Smoothies

"If life gives you lemons, make some kind of fruity juice."
~ Conan O'Brien

Like so many topics related to health and diet, there remains debate over whether juices and smoothies are good for you and, if so, which is better. Many of the plant-based doctors that I follow believe that foods should be chewed, since that starts the digestive process, and they are not proponents of juicing or making smoothies. My personal belief, based on my own experiences only, is that there is a time and place for both.

ჯ

It's important to note that juices and smoothies are two different things. I know many people who use the terms interchangeably, but there is a clear difference. One has pulp; the other does not. Juicing extracts the pulp from the fruits and vegetables to provide only the juice to drink. Smoothies are a blend of intact fruits and vegetables yielding a thicker beverage.

So let's start with juicing.

ჯ

Juicing

I started juicing shortly after my cancer diagnosis. I was lucky enough to have a friend who had a juicer that she didn't use anymore, and she gifted it to me. (Nice, right?) I'll be honest that I didn't have a clue how to use it, and it took me a bit of time to figure it out (even *with* instructions!). Once I did, though, it was time to experiment!

The very first thing I juiced was a cucumber cooler that contained carrots, cucumbers, celery, apple and lemon. I experimented with a number of combinations, but this initial recipe would eventually be the basis of what I lovingly call my "kitchen sink" juice because it contained everything but! A super simple recipe to start is simply equal parts carrots and oranges.

Juicing can be a great part of your cancer treatment program and, in fact, the Gerson Therapy program recommends 13 glasses of organic carrot-apple and green-leaf juices daily (see *gerson.org* for more information). The benefits of juicing, especially during my chemotherapy, were many. The surge of nutrients from the juice helped support my immune system and my gut health. The juice helped me get nutrients from foods that I might have had trouble eating during chemo. It helped with hydration, a long-term issue for me, and I had more energy.

Juicing became a daily ritual for my son and me; we juiced every day after school. He loved the taste and spoke of feeling better himself. He even put together lists of foods you *can* juice, foods you *shouldn't* juice, and foods that mush. Even though we don't juice as often anymore, he'll still ask for it if he starts to feel even the tiniest bit sick. He still swears by its healing properties!

While there are a number of pros to drinking juices, there are some cons as well. The first challenge is that juicing does require a special machine. I was lucky to have been given one, but they can have quite a wide range in price. The juicer I have is around $100 or so, and I'm not sure I would have spent the money early on, because I wouldn't have known. I'm enormously grateful for the gift, since the juicing did provide a lot of benefits.

For me, the second issue was clean up. After you peel/prep your fruits and veggies for processing, you then need to disassemble the juicer and clean each piece. It's just one of those things that's a pain, even though not necessarily difficult. Part of clean up includes figuring out what to do with all the pulp you extracted. Some people compost it; other, more ambitious people, save it to put in muffins or some other dish. And still others, like me, end up throwing it out. Yes, it does feel wasteful, but since I was going through cancer treatment at the time, I gave myself a pass.

Juicing can be expensive because of the amount of produce you use, and it is recommended that you use organic produce. It's also best to drink it the same day you make it for the best nutritional value, so you can't really make a big batch and save it too long.

If you are watching your sugar intake, you need to be especially careful with juices, as you get all the sugars without the fiber to help slow absorption. It's always best to use more vegetables than fruits to help keep the sugar content lower.

ጸ

Michele's "Kitchen Sink" Juice

>   8 carrots
>   1 English cucumber
>   2-3 stalks of celery
>   1 apple
>   1-2 oranges
>   1" piece of ginger root
>   Whatever else you might want to add, including: strawberries, red beets, pears, etc.
>   Push all fruits and vegetables through the juicer. Stir and pour over ice. Enjoy!

ጸ

Smoothies

These beverages are made by pureeing fruits and vegetables. They may also be blended with yogurt, coconut water, various types of milk, ice, and sweeteners.

Similar to juices, smoothies are a delicious way to get some extra veggies into your diet and work really well with children. It's a great way to hide greens, especially! The advantage smoothies have over juices is that they contain all the fiber from the fruits and veggies you are including. The fiber helps to slow absorption of the fructose and nutrients. Drinking smoothies may help with your weight loss efforts if you are using them as a meal replacement and it may help with digestion since the blender is, in effect, pre-chewing your food for you.

Another benefit is the ease of preparing smoothies and cleaning up. There is no special machine required; you can make smoothies with a standard blender, food processor, ninja, etc.

There are, as with most things, some cons to smoothies. It is always best to chew your own foods, so you are bypassing that step, and it's possible that you end up consuming more calories than if you ate the whole food. If purchasing smoothies from a vendor or restaurant, be sure to ask the ingredients and calorie count. You may think you are doing something healthy, but in actuality may be consuming a high number of calories, fat and sugar, depending on what they add.

I have never been a huge smoothie maker. When I did make them, I tended to start with a good quality plant-protein smooth mix, and then added a banana or a handful of berries for flavor. There are certainly mixed reviews on doing this since the protein mix isn't really a "whole food", but they did help me with my weight loss since they were filling and nutritious. It's just not something I would recommend on a daily basis. Whole foods are always the better option.

$$\text{\r{R}}$$

Whether you juice or make smoothies really comes down to personal preference and where you are with your own health issues. For me, the juices were a critical part of my health regimen during treatment, and smoothies helped me with weight and nutrients. These days, however, I rarely do either. In part, it's because I don't think I need that extra boost because I eat so well. But, admittedly, the juicing fell by the wayside because of the effort involved, and because I got sick of having that big juicer on my counter. That's not to say that I don't still believe they have their place. I think if you are in treatment, and/or you are trying to progress towards eating a healthier diet, I would recommend it. You just may not need it long term, and always be aware of the cautions noted above.

CHAPTER 11

Healing Your Body: Supplementation

*"Well, we all age, but I'd been taking herbal supplements
for a long time." ~Frankie Avalon [57]*

Another topic of debate when it comes to health is
supplementation (vitamins, minerals, herbals). Are they helpful or
hurtful? Are they a good investment or a waste of money? Can
you trust them? Depending on who you ask, you will likely get a
different answer.

I probably fall somewhere in the middle of the spectrum: I don't
think a multi-vitamin is necessary if you are eating a varied,
healthy diet, but I did, and still do, take a number of herbal
supplements to support my overall health. Food is always the best
source for nutrients, since all the nutrients work together; rarely is
it about just one nutrient. (For example, vitamin C by itself versus
vitamin C combined with all the other good stuff in an orange.) At
times, however, we need a little help either because our diets are
missing something or because our bodies are somehow impaired.
It's important to note, however, that no amount of
supplementation can make up for a poor diet. If you are eating the
Standard American Diet but taking a multi-vitamin, it might be
worth re-thinking that.

ช

My first word of advice on this topic is that you find a practitioner
qualified to help you in this process. I certainly don't recommend
taking things willy-nilly as you find them in the dollar store or
some super store. Quality matters, as does getting the appropriate
recommendations on what to take.

I was lucky enough to already be working with a Certified Natural Health Professional when I was diagnosed and she was a great support to me during treatment. She was well qualified with a Bachelor of Science, a certified Natural Health Practitioner from the Trinity School of Natural Health, and a certified iridologist. She has 20+ years of experience in helping people to wellness, and I had/have enormous trust in her.

I highly recommend that you look for someone with this type of experience to help support you in your health journey – especially if you are going through treatment. Her recommendations helped keep me strong and were a great complement to the traditional treatments I was undertaking. Since the exact combination of skills and experience I mentioned above may not exist elsewhere, the best thing to do is to search for a naturopath or natural health practitioner. In order to find someone reputable, you can ask around at health food stores, yoga studios, chiropractors, and friends and family. Your practitioner should be a good example of health and if s/he is not, they probably aren't very good at healing others. (A true statement for traditional medical doctors, as well.)

ጸ

Following is a variety of supplements that I took over the course of my cancer treatment and afterwards, to support my immunity, keep my digestive tract healthy, to balance my hormones, and to help with overall wellness.

It's important to remember that all supplements are not created equally. Do your homework, as always, to ensure that you are getting a quality product. Look at information such as the distributor; if it's from China, I'd be leery. Consider the price. If it sounds too good (cheap) to be true, it probably is. You want to know that if it says "red beet root" on the label, that you aren't getting something else – or worse, filler and chemicals.

- **Vitamin D(D3)**
  I was surprised to learn that Vitamin D isn't a vitamin at all; it's a hormone! [58] Vitamin D helps your body absorb calcium and may help support mood, cardiovascular health, and immunity. Vitamin D is primarily produced by the body from a chemical reaction that occurs when sunlight hits your skin. [59] But if you live in an area where there isn't a lot of sun (like Northeastern

Pennsylvania!), or you aren't much of an outdoors person, chances are that you aren't getting enough Vitamin D. I take Vitamin D pretty much every day, unless it's a summer day, with lots of sun, and I plan to be outside (which doesn't happen much where I live; I should probably say I take it every day - period.)

- **B-12 / Methyl B-12**
  Since I am a vegetarian, B-12 is a vitamin that I'm not getting in my diet, so this is something that I take every day also. B vitamins support the immune and nervous systems and help buffer the effects of stress. Methylated B12 is the best form as it's easier for the liver to process. If you have the activated MTHFR gene, Methyl B-12 is what should be taken to help detox your liver more efficiently. [60]

- **Indole-3-Carbinol**
  Indole-3-Carbinol is a substance formed when cruciferous vegetables are cut, chewed, or cooked. As discussed earlier, cruciferous vegetables are great cancer fighters and should be part of a healthy diet. But if at high risk of cancer or a recurrence, this supplement can be added. I took this during my cancer treatment but no longer take it.

- **E-Tea (Essiac tea formula)**
  The story of Essiac tea is a fascinating one, and I recommend that you search for the story online for more information. This tea was developed by a Canadian nurse, Rene Caisse, in the early 1900s and was used to heal cancer patients. (Essiac is Caisse spelled backwards.) She fought an uphill battle to bring this formula into the mainstream but was fighting against conventional wisdom, politics, and money. While not FDA approved, Essiac tea can be found in many health food stores and is often used by cancer patients. I did not take the tea itself, but rather a supplement made from the ingredients from that formula. Like the Indole-3-Carbinol, I took this during cancer treatment and for a while after, but no longer.

- **Probiotics**
  I am convinced that taking a probiotic during my chemo treatment prevented me for having nausea and diarrhea by keeping my gut bacteria healthy. I continue to take one called Probiotic Eleven on a daily basis, but I took a higher dose during chemo.

- **Aloe Vera Juice**
  In addition to the probiotics, I regularly drank aloe vera juice to help soothe my digestive tract. Another good choice is slippery elm.

- **Iodine**
  I do take iodine daily to help protect my thyroid from likely damage from treatment. Plus, I don't use an iodized salt, so I'm probably not getting enough from my diet. Good sources of iodine include kelp, potassium iodide, or black walnut. Low levels of iodine are linked with breast cancer, as the cells need iodine to fend off tumor growth and kill off the cancer cells. [61]

- **Phosphatidylserine**
  This one was not recommended by my naturalist, but rather by a fellow breast cancer survivor who suggested it for helping my failing memory. I took it for a while but did not find it to be helpful to me. I know others have had success with it, even if I did not.

- **Hormonal Support**
  Let's face it: my hormones are shot. As we discussed earlier in the book, I've got fried ovaries and menopause to contend with! I will forever take *something* to help support my hormones. This is something that I review with my naturalist on a quarterly basis and adjust as necessary. Below is a list of a number of supplements I have taken at various times over the years.

○ **Herbal Estrogens**
   I take a blend of phytoestrogens to help manage menopausal symptoms, like hot flashes. Top herbs in this formula include black cohosh root and dong quai root. Additionally, flaxseed oil or flaxseed meal are a rich source of lignans, a phytoestrogen most similar to human estrogen. [62]

○ **Other Women's Hormones**
   I take a number of other herbals to support various hormones, including progesterone and testosterone. Among the key herbals: maca root extract, l-arginine, licorice root, and DHEA.

○ **Wild Yam, or Wild Yam & Chaste Tree**
   Wild yam is a commonly used herbal for support of female hormones, as a plant based source of progesterone. Chaste tree supports the pituitary gland, where other hormones are produced.

○ **Dulse, Bladderwrack, Kelp**
   These seaweeds help rid your body of the xenoestrogens (or "bad" estrogens) from chemicals or other toxins in the environment. Additionally, they are a great source of iodine.

○ **Other blends**
   There are a number of other blends that I have taken, which include herbals such as red raspberry leaves, blessed thistle, dong quai root, marshmallow root, lobelia, and more. A skilled, experience naturopath or naturalist will be able to help determine which are best for you.

• **Calcium / Calcium-D-Glucarate**
From time to time, I need to take a calcium supplement, but that's usually if I haven't been getting enough leafy greens in my diet. Beans and tofu are also great sources of calcium, but sometimes you still might need a boost. The Calcium-D-Glucarate, more specifically, is used for preventing a variety of cancers, including breast, by helping to remove toxins from the body. [63]

- **Lymph Gland Cleanse**
  This blend of herbals contains parthenium, goldenseal, capsicum and more to support the lymphatic system. Given my periodic flare-ups of lymphedema, this is sometimes needed.

- **Antioxidants**
  Some of the antioxidants I took from time to time to support my immune system include: Pau d'Arco, Una de Gato, Ginger, Turmeric, and green tea.
  I tried Oregano Oil but since I'm not a fan of oregano, I really couldn't tolerate the smell! Very strong!

- **Liquid Chlorophyll**
  This supplement helps your body transport oxygen to your tissues, which has been shown to lower cancer risk. [64]

As you can see, I still try to get all/most of my nutrients from whole foods. It truly is the best source. But sometimes our bodies have had damage or issues that aren't easily solved with food. I think supplementation *where you need it* makes sense. It definitely worked (and still does work) for me.

CHAPTER 12

Healing Your Body: Lifestyle Changes

"Take care of your body. It's the only place you have to live in."
~Jim Rohn [65]

Eating right to nourish your body is so very important, but it's not the only thing you can, and should, do to give yourself the best shot at being cancer free. This chapter will cover a number of other lifestyle changes do improve your odds.

ℛ

Avoid Toxins

When you stop to think about all the places toxins can enter your body, it can be overwhelming. Toxins can exist in what we consume, touch, breathe and think! It's unrealistic to think we can avoid them 100 percent of the time without living in a bubble. However, there are many actions you can take that help to mitigate all the risks we discussed in Chapter 3.

- **Tobacco**
  If you are a smoker or tobacco-chewer, quitting is absolutely the number one thing you should do to improve your health. While cancer risk is the biggest risk to smoking, there are so many other health problems associated with being a smoker: risk of stroke and heart disease, cataracts, hearing loss, asthma and bronchitis, emphysema, slower healing of wounds, lowered fertility, stomach ulcers, and premature wrinkling, to name but a few. [66]

- **Radiation**
  As covered in the chapter on diagnostics, we know that
  excess exposure to radiation can cause cancer. But who
  knows what "excess" means to *your* body? I always
  challenge my doctors for alternatives to any follow up tests
  they require (Do I really need a chest x-ray? Can I have an
  MRI instead of a CT Scan?), as well as the frequency. I
  have pushed back on my dentist, even, when he has
  requested x-rays. It's not that I never do dental x-rays, but
  I do challenge how frequently they need to be done.
  Again, it will depend on your individual situation, but
  don't be afraid to ask.

- **Xenoestrogens**
  Avoid/minimize access to xenoestrogens, which are
  chemicals that disrupt normal functioning of your
  hormones. Many of these xenoestrogens have estrogen-like
  qualities, so frequent access to them may cause an
  overabundance of estrogen (estrogen dominance). These
  excesses are stored in our fat cells and are linked to a
  number of problems, including infertility; obesity;
  endometriosis; and breast, prostate, and testicular cancer.

  Examples of xenoestrogens: birth control pills (ask your
  doctor about alternatives for birth control), pesticides,
  plastics, skin care items, make up, and insecticides.

  Some tips for avoiding xenoestrogens [67]:

    o   Eat organic produce if you can afford it (and if you
        can't, eating conventionally-grown fruits and
        veggies is still better than the alternative). I try to
        specifically buy organic for those items that I
        consume more regularly.
    o   Avoid plastics and especially don't microwave
        your foods in plastic containers. I use glass storage
        containers.
    o   Install a water filter for your drinking water.
    o   Use natural products such as soaps, toothpaste,
        creams and cosmetics; pay attention to what you
        put on your skin.
    o   Use chemical-free cleaning products.

- Avoid noxious smells, such as turning your head away from the pump when you are filling your car's gas tank.
- Switch to an aluminum-free deodorant. While there is much debate on this particular topic, my philosophy is "when in doubt, don't."

- **Alcohol**
Don't overuse alcohol. What does that mean, exactly? According to the National Institutes of Health, too much is related to too much at one time, too frequent, or both. Low-risk drinking for women is defined as no more than three servings of alcohol in a day AND no more than seven a week. For men, the limits are no more than four in a day AND no more than 14 in a week. [68]

In case you are thinking you can just use a bigger glass, it's important to be familiar with what constitutes a serving:

- Beer (regular): 12 oz.
- Beer (malt): 8 oz.
- Wine: 5 oz.
- Cordial/Liqueur: 2-3 oz.
- Brandy: 1.5 oz.
- Distilled spirits: 1.5 oz.

Women who drink, even moderately, have a much greater risk of developing breast cancer than those who abstain – as much as 40-100 percent greater. [69]

- **Other known carcinogens**
The International Agency for Research on Cancer publishes a full list of "known and probable" human carcinogens. I recommend reviewing the list on the American Cancer Society site to see what pertains to you. Depending on where you live, what type of work you perform, etc., some may be more meaningful to you than others. [70]

ॡ

Exercise

Exercise contributes to a lower risk of cancer by helping you manage your weight, strengthening your immune system, and helping to balance hormones and insulin. Particularly, aerobic exercise will help the oxygen flow to tissues and cells, decreasing your risk of cancer. [71]

Admittedly, along with proper hydration, exercise is a challenge for me. I like to do exercise that feels productive in nature. For example, I love to mow the lawn (push mower, of course) and shovel snow. But those are limited opportunities and not nearly enough. Outside of household activities, yoga is probably my favorite exercise, but I am not as consistent as I would like. The treadmill is something else I'll do if I am able to multi-task (watch a video, read a book, write, etc.).

Whatever your favorite exercise (and I'll use the word "favorite" loosely for those of you like me), the important thing is to move. The American Cancer Society recommends 150 minutes of moderate intensity activity per week, OR 75 minutes of vigorous exercise, if so inclined. Moderate intensity can be as simple as walking 3 mph (which is one mile in 20 minutes); 150 minutes a week is only 21 minutes a day, so it's totally doable. [72]

ጸ

Sleep

More and more research is being done on the impact of sleep (or lack thereof) on cancer. Given that your body does a lot of its work on regulating and repairing cells while you sleep, it stands to reason that a chronically-sleep-deprived person might have a higher risk of cancer growth. Sleep is the time your body builds up its immune system and restores cells and DNA. Now, this doesn't mean one night's bad sleep will result in cancer. However, long-term, chronic sleep issues may be one more risk factor. [73]

In the book, *Sleep Smarter*, Shawn Stevenson says that, "There isn't one facet of your mental, emotional, or physical performance that's not affected by the quality of your sleep." [74] The average adult needs at least 7-9 hours of quality sleep for optimal performance. [75] If you are looking for a great resource on how sleep impacts the brain, check out Daniel G. Amen's book, *Change Your Brain Change Your Life.* Both of these resources are excellent if sleep deprivation is a challenge for you.

ጸ

Stress Management

There isn't evidence that stress *causes* cancer, per se. However, there may be a connection to its growth. [76]

Cortisol, the primary stress hormone, is usually self-regulating during fight-or-flight situations, returning to normal levels after the stressful situation is over. Cortisol works to suppress "non-essential" functions during an emergency, such as your immune system. In the short term, this isn't a big deal, but during prolonged periods of stress and unregulated cortisol levels, this suppression may allow chronic illness, such as cancer, to run amok.

I lost a dear friend, a co-worker, to breast cancer a few years ago. She was doing many of the healthy lifestyle and diet changes that I have discussed above. We met regularly to compare notes and to help keep each other on track. She swore that each occurrence of breast cancer was precipitated by a period of extreme stress. Indeed, she was working in a stressful job, working ridiculously long hours, and caring for elderly parents. She absolutely believed that stress played a part.

For me, managing my stress meant making a promise to myself to work manageable hours, to get enough rest, and to just let some things go. I try to find time for fun with family and friends, and to participate in activities that I enjoy. The one thing that cancer is really good at is providing perspective. Once you've had cancer, it's a lot easier to find a balance and to only worry about things that truly matter.

ጸ

I know seems like a lot of changes – diet, exercise, sleeping right, managing stress – and it is. This didn't all happen overnight for me. It took, quite literally, years. It's still a process, if I'm being honest. But they are areas to start working on, a little at a time.

CHAPTER 13

The Cost of Breast Cancer

"Beware of little expenses. A small leak will sink a great ship."
~Benjamin Franklin

I was fortunate to have good medical insurance during my breast cancer treatment. Yet, even with insurance, out-of-pocket expenses quickly added up. After my treatment was done, I went through my financial records to prepare for a speech at a breast cancer charity and I was surprised at just how high the number was: over $8,000! That was for treatment that lasted about eight months (not counting the hormone therapy time) and for which I was covered by insurance.

§

Copayments and coinsurances are payments that the patient/insured must pay to a medical provider as a shared cost of health services or prescription medications. Typically, a co-payment is a flat dollar amount and does not generally apply to your deductible; co-insurance is a percentage of the overall cost after the deductible is met. The deductible is the amount you must pay out of pocket before your insurance pays any claims.

All of the following providers and services that were paid copays and/or coinsurance: gynecologist, surgeon, pathologist, oncologist, radiological oncologist, physical therapist, and occupational therapist. The last two were due to my lymphedema.

I also had co-payments for blood/lab work, x-rays, CT scans, and prescriptions (steroids, antibiotics, anti-nausea drugs). My copayment for each Neulasta shot alone was $100 – and I needed six of those over the course of my treatment. At the time, I was advised that these shots cost $3600 without insurance, which is just insane.

And, of course, because my treatment crossed plan years, I had to meet my deductible a second time at the start of the new year.

ᘒ

As I have mentioned previously, I saw a naturalist regularly during my treatment. Those appointments and all of my supplements were not covered by insurance.

ᘒ

The $8000+ number also did *NOT* include:

- **Wig**
  My wig ($300) was not covered by insurance and was never worn beyond the first week. Some insurance plans may cover this, so always check. If it does *not*, really think about it before you invest the money. You may also be able to find places that donate wigs to women battling cancer.

- **Scarves**
  I ended up with a pretty nice collection of scarves, in every color of the rainbow, plain and patterned. This is what I wore every day and they were worth every penny. They were about $20-25 each, so I did invest some big bucks here, but I was glad I did. They have been worn by at least four other cancer warriors, so they have paid for themselves several times over.

- **New clothing**
  My wonderful friends bought me a number of new tops and pajamas to get through my treatment and beyond. But after all was said and done, I needed to take a good look at my closet. My shape was forever changed and some clothing just wasn't going to work anymore. Since I worked in Corporate America at the time, I did invest in some new clothing that was more suited for my breast-less body.

- **Over-the-counter medications**
  I used Tylenol for minor pain and headaches, Claritin for leg cramps, and Mucinex when my low immunity got me sick.

77

- **Mouthwash**
  It was recommended that I purchase a special mouthwash for mouth sores that it was expected I would get during chemo. I never did get any sores, so I could have saved my money on this one. Not that it was the worse of my expenses, but every dollar adds up.

- **Electric razor**
  This was suggested because of the risk of cuts and infection during chemo. In retrospect, this was a silly purchase. Since you typically lose your hair during chemo, why would you ever need one of these? Face palm!

- **Lotions** for my skin during radiation

- **Compression shirts** to help manage my lymphedema. My husband found a great sale at the local outlet, or these would have cost us a lot more than they did.

- **Hearing Aid**
  Related to my hearing loss from nerve damage, I needed a hearing aid. Thankfully, it was only one, as the cost was $3,700! Unfortunately, hearing aids are apparently considered a luxury or cosmetic item – or as they call them, "elective" – as most insurance companies do not cover the cost. I found that to be absolutely infuriating.

&

One last thing not included in the $8,000+ – the generosity of family and friends. While not a direct out-of-pocket expense for us, there is an additional cost to those who love us. Pre-surgery lunches, home-cooked meals, snacks, gifts, clothes, movies, books, cash – the generosity cannot be calculated. The most important commodity? Time spent, which is invaluable.

CHAPTER 14

Learn More

"Education is the most powerful weapon we can use to change the world..."~Nelson Mandela [77]

I'm a big believer in knowledge as a driver of behavioral changes. The more you know, the more you can challenge conventional wisdom, ask the right questions, and understand what changes you need to make – and *WHY* you need to make them.

When I was starting my health journey, I didn't really know where to start. But what was important was to just *start*. Pick up a book. Just start somewhere, anywhere. That one book will lead you to another and another and another. If you don't like to read, watch a documentary – or two or three or more!

Learn and evolve your behaviors like your life depended on it, because it does.

Ⴟ

Following is a list of my favorite books, documentaries, and websites. There are thousands more resources to tap into, but this is a great starting point.

Books
My Top Picks:

- *Crazy Sexy Diet: Eat Your Veggies, Ignite Your Spark, and Live Like You Mean It!*, by Kris Carr
This was the book that started it all for me! I am forever grateful for that magazine article all those years ago that led me to this book, and to Kris Carr, for sharing her journey to health. For most people, I recommend starting with this book just because it's a lighter read, often humorous, and it just makes so much damn sense!

- *The China Study: The Most Comprehensive Study of Nutrition Ever Conducted and the Startling Implications for Diet, Weight Loss and Long-term Health,* by T. Colin Campbell, PhD, with Thomas M. Campbell II
If you are interested in preventing, reversing, or healing from cancer, this book demonstrates the link between animal protein and cancer based on years of research by Dr. Campbell and his teams. I credit Dr. Campbell with saving my life with this book, and I was so excited to meet him at a conference and get his autograph. He is a rock star of plant-based nutrition!

- *The Starch Solution: Eat the Foods You Love, Regain Your Health, and Lose the Weight for Good!*, John A. McDougall and Mary McDougall
There are many variations on a plant-based diet theme. This is the one that I ended up following and it helps you see that carbs are not evil. In fact, they are enormously healthful. We have maligned the poor potato, but Dr. McDougall shows you how a potato (and other starch)-filled diet can improve your health and reverse disease.

- *How Not to Die: Discover the Foods Scientifically Proven to Prevent and Reverse Disease*, by Michael Greger, MD and Gene Stone
If you are looking for the science behind plant-based nutrition, and if you need the studies to prove it to yourself, this is the book for you, with over 100 pages of studies cited. I found this to just be a fascinating read, regardless of your health or diagnosis, and this was the book that convinced me to add soy to my diet.

- *Keep It Simple, Keep It Whole: Your Guide to Optimum Health* by Alona Pulde, MD, and Matthew Lederman, MD
  I love the food continuum in this book and the way they assign a grade to your existing diet and teach you how to improve that grade. For example, if your diet is presently an "F" (processed, fried, and fast foods), then you probably want to first improve your grade to a "D" before trying to jump to an "A+".

- *Dr. Neal Barnard's Program for Reversing Diabetes: The Scientifically Proven System for Reversing Diabetes Without Drugs,* by Dr. Neal Barnard and Bryanna Clark-Grogan, and *Prevent and Reverse Heart Disease,* by Dr. Caldwell B. Esselstyn, Jr.
  While my book is about cancer, I wanted to include these last two books on diabetes and heart disease. Very often, chronic diseases come in multiples because they are all often coming from the same source: poor diet and lifestyle choices that lead to inflammation that, in turn, lead to disease. Helping one helps all.

Other great choices:

- *Chris Beat Cancer: A Comprehensive Plan for Healing Naturally,* by Chris Wark

- *Whole: Rethinking the Science of Nutrition,* by T. Colin Campbell, Ph.D. with Howard Jacobson, Ph.D.
  I have this one autographed, too! Read *The China Study* first, since this one is a bit more scientific and heavier.

- *Anticancer: A New Way of Life,* by David Servan-Schreiber, M.D., Ph.D.

- *The Cancer Survivor's Guide: Foods that help you fight back!* by Neal D. Barnard, M.D., Jennifer K. Reilly, R.D., and Susan M. Levin, M.S., R.D.

- *Foods to Fight Cancer: What To Eat to Reduce Your Risk,* by Richard Beliveau, Ph.D. and Dr. Denis Gingras

- *The 9 Steps To Keep the Doctor Away: Simple Actions to Shift Your Body and Mind to Optimum Health for Greater Longevity*, by Dr. Rashid A. Buttar

- *Knockout: Interviews With Doctors Who Are Curing Cancer — And How to Prevent Getting It In the First Place*, by Suzanne Somers

- *The Cheese Trap: How Breaking a Surprising Addiction Will Help You Lose Weight, Gain Energy, and Get Healthy*, by Dr. Neal Barnard

- *Sleep Smarter: 21 Essential Strategies to Sleep Your Way to a Better Body, Better Health, and Bigger Success*, by Shawn Stevenson

ࠚ

Cookbooks and Recipe Sites:

Here is a list of some of my favorite cookbooks. Note that several of these include recipes with oil. If you are transitioning to a healthier diet with more plants, you may choose to use the oil initially. I almost always just eliminate the oil with zero impact on the recipe. If there is sautéing involved, I simply use a bit of veggie broth instead of the oil.

- *Isa Does It: Amazingly Easy, Wildly Delicious Vegan Recipes for Every Day of the Week,* by Isa Chandra Moskowitz
  I probably use this cookbook vastly more than any other. Its pages are well-worn and well-stained!

- *Vegan With a Vengeance Cookbook: Over 150 Delicious, Cheap, Animal-Free Recipes That Rock*, by Isa Chandra Moskowitz

- *How Not to Die Cookbook: Over 100 Recipes to Help Prevent and Reverse Disease*, by Michael Greger, MD, FACLM, with Gene Stone, recipes by Robin Robertson

- *The Oh She Glows Cookbook: Over 100 Vegan Recipes to Glow from the Inside Out*, by Angela Liddon

- *Chloe's Kitchen: 125 Easy, Delicious Recipes for Making the Food You Love the Vegan Way*, by Chloe Coscarelli

- *The 40-Year-Old Vegan: 75 Recipes to Make You Leaner, Cleaner, and Greener in the Second Half of Life*, by Sandra Sellani and Susan Sellani

- *McDougall Quick and Easy Cookbook: Over 300 Delicious Low-Fat Recipes You Can Prepare in Fifteen Minutes or Less*, by John A. McDougall, M.D., and Mary McDougall

- *The Happy Herbivore Cookbook*, by Lindsay S. Nixon

- *Happy Herbivore Light & Lean*, by Lindsay S. Nixon

- *The Engine 2 Cookbook: More than 130 Lip-Smacking, Rib-Sticking, Body-Slimming Recipes to Live Plant Strong*, by Rip Esselstyn and Jane Esselstyn
  This one is a great resource for the men in your life, since Rip Esselstyn was a Texas firefighter.

- *The Vegan 8: 100 Simple, Delicious Recipes Made with 8 Ingredients or Less*, by Brandi Doming

- *Minimalist Baker's Everyday Cooking*, by Dana Shultz

- *The Anti-Breast Cancer Cookbook: How to Cut Your Risk with the Most Powerful, Cancer-Fighting Foods*, by Julia B. Greer, M.D., MPH

- *Crazy Sexy Kitchen: 150 Plant-Empowered Recipes to Ignite a Mouthwatering Revolution*, by Kris Carr with Chef Chad Sarno

- *The China Study Cookbook*, by LeAnne Campbell

- *The Cancer Survivor's Guide: Foods that help you fight back*, by Neal D Barnard, M.D., and Jennifer K Reilly, R.D.

- *HappyHerbivore.com*
  Lindsay Nixon's cookbooks were some of the first I used when I was starting a plant-based diet. Her website includes access to her blog, tips on getting started, and a recipes section. She also offers meal plans on her site that may be helpful when you are starting out and unsure of what to cook.

There are hundreds (if not thousands) of plant-based recipe websites to search for recipes that fit your palate. You can also use your favorite search engine to find a healthier version of your favorite meat-based meal(s) – just add the word "vegan. For example: "vegan lasagna"! And let's not forget Pinterest. While I am not a very good Pinterest user myself, I know many people who find great recipes on this site and have figured out how to "pin" and manage those recipes. (I think I need a class!)

ቶ

Documentaries

Many of these documentaries can be found on Netflix, Amazon Prime, and/or YouTube.

- *Forks Over Knives*
  This should be the first one on your watch list!
- *What the Health*
- *The C Word*
- *Eating You Alive*
- *Food Matters*
- *Hungry for Change*
- *Plant Pure Nation*
- *Vegucated*
- *Fat, Sick & Nearly Dead*
- *Food, Inc.*
- *Cowspiracy*

ቶ

Websites/Blogs

- *LightsCancerAction.wordpress.com* and *MetamorphosisMindBodySpirit.com*
  These two links are both my personal sites. The first is my blog page where I chronicled my breast cancer journey from diagnosis through treatment and beyond. The second is my health coaching website and contains a lot of helpful information including a library of my favorite plant-based recipes, additional blog materials, and contact information. You can also find a description of the services I offer and my approach to health coaching.

- *ForksOverKnives.com*
  Aligned with the documentary and other FOK resources, the website is a great place to go to get all your plant-based questions answered. They also have a huge recipe library (already "no oil") and corresponding recipe app for your phone.

- *DrMcDougall.com*
  This site supports *The Starch Solution* plant-based diet. You can get access to prior newsletters, enroll in Dr. McDougall's programs in Santa Rosa, California, and access a wide variety of informational articles. This site has a discussion board for you to connect with others struggling with a particular illness, a recipe section, and one of my favorite documents for sharing: Dr. McDougall's Color Picture Book. In the simplest of terms – red, yellow, and green foods – it is made clear what you should and should not eat.

- *NutritionFacts.org*
  This site is run by Dr. Michael Greger (of *How Not to Die* fame) and contains thousands of videos (and transcripts) pertaining to plant-based nutrition and how it benefits many diseases. As with his book, the website contains all the supporting science. It is my first stop with any research I may be doing.

- *PCRM.org*
  The Physicians Committee for Responsible Medicine is a group of thousands of physicians dedicated to improving the health of people and animals through plant-based nutrition and ethical scientific research. Their site has a lot of great resources.

- *Gerson.org*
  I referenced Gerson Therapy in the juicing section earlier. You can find out more about their alternative treatment program on this site.

- *KrisCarr.com*
  You can sign up for a newsletter with periodic motivation and support. The site also contains a recipe section and a number of other sections for overall health. Her blog has a number of tips specific to cancer prevention.

- *ChrisBeatCancer.com*
  Diagnosed with Stage IIIc colon cancer, Chris opted out of chemo and healed himself with nutrition and natural therapies. He's got a ton of great resources, including a book, a website, videos, testimonials, and more.

- *Facebook Groups*
  You can also find hundreds of different support groups on Facebook. Some are more militant than others, so if you aren't finding the right support for you, move on to another group.

The Internet is your friend! You can find all the resources you need to get started – for free!

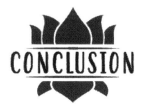

CONCLUSION

*"It's the possibility that keeps me going, not the guarantee,
a sort of wager on my part." ~Nicholas Sparks, The Notebook [78]*

Mine is just one story out of millions of stories – millions of women who have dealt, or are dealing, with breast cancer. Many of us have made it to the other side, but far too many have not. For those of us doing ok, the fear of a recurrence is always near.

One in eight women will develop breast cancer in her lifetime. Think about your circle of friends – 1 in 8. Who will it be next?

While death rates have been decreasing for the past few decades, an estimated 41,000 women died of breast cancer in 2018.

The National Cancer Institute estimates that about $500-600 *million* goes into breast cancer research each year. [79] That's a lot of money and, although rates of deaths are declining, 41,000 deaths are 41,000 too many. While we invest in finding a cure, perhaps we can and should take matters into our own hands. While nothing is a guarantee, wouldn't you want to try everything you could to stay healthy? To not get breast cancer? To not die prematurely?

I hope this book has given you some inspiration to make some changes in your own life, whether you have been diagnosed with breast cancer or not. My journey has been easier than many, and yet I have more than my fair share of scars from the battle. There's no one right answer for everyone, but I urge you to listen to your body. It is speaking to you all the time. It speaks through temperatures and scales, through bowel movements and energy levels, through pain and hunger cues. What is your body telling you? What is it asking for? What does it need to heal?

Listen. Then act.

No guarantees, but great possibility.

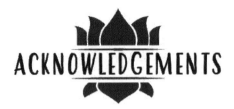

ACKNOWLEDGEMENTS

Very few things happen in a vacuum, and writing a book is certainly no exception to that. While this book is *my* health journey, I did not walk that path alone. I owe a debt of gratitude to all of those people who took the journey with me, and those who supported me in the writing of this book. I don't know how I can possibly repay you!

᪥

To the hundreds of family members, friends, health care providers, coworkers, and neighbors who supported me during my breast cancer diagnosis, treatment, and health journey – I would not be here without you.

To Leann Yannuzzi, "my Leann", thank you for agreeing to be my accountability coach on this book and for sharing your feedback throughout the writing process. You have been there for so many critical events in my life; you have been my rock through so much these past 20+ years. How would I have ever coped without you in my life?

Aimee Long, Certified Natural Health Professional, healer extraordinaire, and friend: You were the first to highlight issues with my right breast, about one year before actually being diagnosed! You have kept me strong through treatment and have balanced my hormones ever since. I am grateful for your contributions to this book and for helping me to keep my supplements straight!

Many thanks to my editor and friend, Sheryl Sochoka. There is no one whose editing and honesty I trust more! Thank you for making time for me, even when your own life was hectic. Thank you, also, for saving me on the book cover "optimization"; that was well beyond my comprehension or skills!

To my many proofreaders – family and friends whose recommendations and feedback were invaluable to the quality of the final product: Dyanne Potter Voegtlin, Marissa Yannuzzi, Dr. Burns, David Orrson, Sheryl Sochoka, Aimee Long, Dessa Tripus, and Sandra Tripus. I am so grateful for all of the time and energy you put into this project. Your faith in me seemed unshakeable, and I am forever humbled by all you have done for me. Marissa, a special thanks for your support on citations and Photoshop layers!

Thank you to the many of you who encouraged me to write a book over the years. There are too many of you to list, but I am grateful for your trust and faith.

The resources at the Institute of Integrative Nutrition have been amazing. I would never have figured this self-publishing, book-writing thing out on my own. They have been so responsive to every question and knowledgeable about every nuance of writing a book.

Lastly, thank you to my husband, David, and son, Ethan, who have been somewhat neglected while I wrote. Thank you for making adjustments in your lives to allow me to pursue a new career and this dream of mine. Thank you, always, for your love.

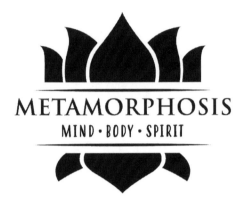

metamorphosismindbodyspirit.com

lightscanceraction.wordpress.com

metamorphosismindbodyspirit@gmail.com

Michele Tripus Orrson

Integrative Nutrition Health Coach

Certified in Plant Based Nutrition from
T. Colin Campbell Center for Nutrition Studies and eCornell

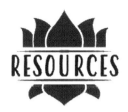

RESOURCES

Notes

[1] Pasha, Riz. "109 Greatest Zig Ziglar Quotes Of All Time - Succeed Feed". *Succeed Feed*, https://succeedfeed.com/zig-ziglar-quotes/.

[2] "Dictionary By Merriam-Webster: America's Most-Trusted Online Dictionary". *Merriam-Webster.Com*, 2019, https://www.merriam-webster.com/dictionary/.

[3] "Invasive Lobular Carcinoma - Symptoms And Causes". *Mayo Clinic*, 2018, https://www.mayoclinic.org/diseases-conditions/invasive-lobular-carcinoma/symptoms-causes/syc-20373973.

[4] "Tests For Diagnosing ILC". *Breastcancer.Org*, 2016, https://www.breastcancer.org/symptoms/types/ilc/tests/diagnosing.

[5] "Types Of Breast Cancer: Non-Invasive, Invasive And More". *Breastcancer.Org*, 2018, https://www.breastcancer.org/symptoms/types.

[6] "Stage 2:: The National Breast Cancer Foundation". *Www.Nationalbreastcancer.Org*, 2016, https://www.nationalbreastcancer.org/breast-cancer-stage-2.

[7] "What Are The Stages Of Breast Cancer?". *WebMD*, https://www.webmd.com/breast-cancer/guide/stages-breast-cancer#1.

[8] "Staging". *National Cancer Institute*, 2015, https://www.cancer.gov/about-cancer/diagnosis-staging/staging.

[9] "Grades And Stages". *Breast Cancer Now*, 2016, https://breastcancernow.org/about-breast-cancer/have-you-recently-been-diagnosed-with-breast-cancer/understanding-your-results/grades-and-stages.

[10] "Types Of Breast Cancer: ER-Positive, HER2-Positive, And Triple Negative". *WebMD*, https://www.webmd.com/breast-cancer/guide/breast-cancer-types-er-positive-her2-positive#1.

[11] U.S. Senate Special Committee on Aging (2014) (Testimony of Valerie Harper).

[12] "Tests For Diagnosing ILC". *Breastcancer.Org*, 2016, https://www.breastcancer.org/symptoms/types/ilc/tests/diagnosing.

[13] Greger, FACLM, Michael. "Can Mammogram Radiation Cause Breast Cancer? | Nutritionfacts.Org". *Nutritionfacts.Org*, 2018, https://nutritionfacts.org/video/Can-Mammogram-radiation-Cause-Breast-Cancer/.

[14] Narod, S A et al. "Impact of screening mammography on mortality from breast cancer before age 60 in women 40 to 49 years of age" Current oncology (Toronto, Ont.) vol. 21,5 (2014): 217-21.

[15] "Why Mammography Screening Is Being Abolished In Switzerland | Thermography Center Of Sonoma County". *Thermography-Sc.Com*, 2017, http://www.thermography-sc.com/why-mammography-screening-is-being-abolished-in-switzerland/.

[16] Halls, MD, FRCPC, Steven B. "When To Use MRI For Breast Cancer Screening - Moose And Doc". *Breast Cancer - Moose And Doc*, 2019, https://breast-cancer.ca/mri-how-when/.

[17] Brown, Ken. "Ultrasound For Breast Cancer Diagnosis: Johns Hopkins Breast Center". *Hopkinsmedicine.Org*, https://www.hopkinsmedicine.org/breast_center/treatments_services/breast_cancer_diagnosis/breast_ultrasound.html.

[18] "Ultrasound | Breastcancer.Org". Breastcancer.Org, 2015, https://www.breastcancer.org/symptoms/testing/types/ultrasound.

[19] "What Is Breast Thermography". *Breastthermography.Com*, 2016, http://www.breastthermography.com/breast_thermography_mf.htm.

[20] Brown, Ken. "Breast Biopsy For Breast Cancer Diagnosis: Johns Hopkins Breast Center". *Hopkinsmedicine.Org*, https://www.hopkinsmedicine.org/breast_center/treatments_services/breast_cancer_diagnosis/breast_biopsy.html.

[21] "Stages And Differentiation Of Cancer - All About Cancer". *All About Cancer*, https://www.allaboutcancer.fi/facts-about-cancer/stages/.

[22] Mayo Clinic Staff. "Breast Cancer - Diagnosis And Treatment - Mayo Clinic". *Mayoclinic.Org*, https://www.mayoclinic.org/diseases-conditions/breast-cancer/diagnosis-treatment/drc-20352475.

[23] Snicket, Lemony. *The Slippery Slope*. Harpercollins, 2012.

[24] "Genetics". *National Cancer Institute*, 2017, https://www.cancer.gov/about-cancer/causes-prevention/genetics.

[25] "Study: Five Healthy Habits Lower Cancer Risk". *American Institute For Cancer Research*, 2018, http://www.aicr.org/cancer-research-update/2018/1-24/experts-tout-healthy-lifestyle-is-better-than-any-pill.html.

[26] "Breast Cancer Risk Factors Table". *Ww5.Komen.Org*, 2018, https://ww5.komen.org/Breastcancer/Breastcancerriskfactorstable.html.

[27] "What's Low-Risk Drinking? - Rethinking Drinking - NIAAA". *Rethinkingdrinking.NIAAA.NIH.Gov*, https://www.rethinkingdrinking.niaaa.nih.gov/How-much-is-too-much/Is-your-drinking-pattern-risky/Whats-Low-Risk-Drinking.aspx.

[28] "Eating Unhealthy Food". *Breastcancer.Org*, https://www.breastcancer.org/risk/factors/unhealthy_food.

[29] "Smoking And Breast Cancer Risk". Breastcancer.Org, https://www.breastcancer.org/risk/factors/smoking.

[30] "Breast Cancer Risk Factors Table". *Ww5.Komen.Org*, 2018, https://ww5.komen.org/Breastcancer/Breastcancerriskfactorstable.html.

[31] Bollinger, Ty. "Is There A Connection Between Antibiotic Use And Cancer?". *The Truth About Cancer*, 2018, https://thetruthaboutcancer.com/connection-antibiotic-use-cancer/.

[32] Mayo Clinic Staff. "Sentinel Node Biopsy - Mayo Clinic". *Mayoclinic.Org*, https://www.mayoclinic.org/tests-procedures/sentinel-node-biopsy/about/pac-20385264.

[33] Keller, Julia. "The Mysterious Ambrose Redmoon's Healing Words". *Chicago Tribune*, 2002, https://www.chicagotribune.com/news/ct-xpm-2002-03-29-0203290018-story.html. Accessed 21 Feb 2019.

[34] "Hiccups". *Cancer.Org*, 2015, https://www.cancer.org/treatment/treatments-and-side-effects/physical-side-effects/hiccups.html.

[35] Mayo Clinic Staff. "Chemo Brain - Symptoms And Causes". *Mayo Clinic*, 2018, https://www.mayoclinic.org/diseases-conditions/chemo-brain/symptoms-causes/syc-20351060.

[36] *The Journal Of NIH Research*, 2, 30, 1990.

[37] "Radiation Therapy". *National Cancer Institute*, 2019, https://www.cancer.gov/about-cancer/treatment/types/radiation-therapy.

[38] Cahalan, Susannah. "The Secret Forces That Are Making You Stressed, Hungry And Sexy". *Nypost.Com*, 2018, https://nypost.com/2018/07/07/the-secret-forces-that-are-making-you-stressed-hungry-and-sexy/.

[39] "Hormone Therapy For Breast Cancer | American Cancer Society". *Cancer.Org*, 2017, https://www.cancer.org/cancer/breast-cancer/treatment/hormone-therapy-for-breast-cancer.html.

[40] "What Are Hormones And What Do They Do? | Hormone Health". *Hormone.Org*, https://www.hormone.org/hormones-and-health/hormones/hormones-and-what-do-they-do.

[41] Franks, ND, Olivia A. M., and Jonathan V. Wright, MD. "Estriol: Its Weakness Is Its Strength | Life Extension Magazine". *Lifeextension.Com*, 2008, https://www.lifeextension.com/magazine/2008/8/Estriol-Its-Weakness-is-its-Strength/Page-01.

[42] Petersen, RPh, CNP, Carol. "Vaginal Use Of Estriol | Women's International Pharmacy". *Women's International Pharmacy*, 2018, https://www.womensinternational.com/vaginal-use-of-estriol/.

[43] McDougall, John A. *Dr. Mcdougall's Digestive Tune-Up*. Healthy Living Publications, 2006, p. x.

[44] "Eating Unhealthy Food". *Breastcancer.Org*, https://www.breastcancer.org/risk/factors/unhealthy_food.

[45] "World Health Organization Says Processed Meat Causes Cancer". *Cancer.Org*, 2015, https://www.cancer.org/latest-news/world-health-organization-says-processed-meat-causes-cancer.html.

[46] Imatome-Yun, Naomi. "Can We Eat To Starve Cancer? [VIDEO]". *Forks Over Knives*, 2015, https://www.forksoverknives.com/cancer-diet-therapy-video/#gs.hWsxXZwH.

[47] "Chemicals In Meat Cooked At High Temperatures And Cancer Risk". *National Cancer Institute*, 2017, https://www.cancer.gov/about-cancer/causes-prevention/risk/diet/cooked-meats-fact-sheet.

[48] Wigmore, Ann. *The Hippocrates Diet And Health Program*. Avery Pub. Group, 1983, p. 9.

[49] Greger, MD, FACLM, Michael. "Meat Industry Response To Meat Being Labeled Carcinogenic | Nutritionfacts.Org". *Nutritionfacts.Org*, 2018, https://nutritionfacts.org/2018/10/11/meat-industry-response-to-meat-being-labeled-carcinogenic/.

[50] "Known And Probable Human Carcinogens". *Cancer.Org*, https://www.cancer.org/cancer/cancer-causes/general-info/known-and-probable-human-carcinogens.html.

[51] https://www.drmcdougall.com/health/education/health-science/common-health-problems/obesity/

[52] Patz, Aviva. "Https://Www.Health.Com". *Health*, 2016, https://www.health.com/nutrition/how-much-protein-per-day.

[53] Cronkleton, Emily. "What Happens If You Eat Too Much Protein?". *Healthline*, https://www.healthline.com/health/too-much-protein#risks.

[54] "Antioxidants". *Betterhealth.Vic.Gov.Au*, https://www.betterhealth.vic.gov.au/health/healthyliving/antioxidants.

[55] Greger, MD, FACLM, Michael. "The Benefits Of Soy | Nutritionfacts.Org". *Nutritionfacts.Org*, 2017, https://nutritionfacts.org/audio/the-benefits-of-soy/.

[56] Greger, MD, FACLM, Michael. "Soy & Breast Cancer | Nutritionfacts.Org". *Nutritionfacts.Org*, 2008, https://nutritionfacts.org/video/soy-breast-cancer-3/.

[57] "Search Results". *Brainyquote*, https://www.brainyquote.com/

[58] "Vitamin D | Hormone Health Network". *Hormone.Org*, https://www.hormone.org/hormones-and-health/hormones/vitamin-d.

[59] "Vitamin D | You And Your Hormones From The Society For Endocrinology". *Yourhormones.Info*, 2018, http://www.yourhormones.info/hormones/vitamin-d/.

[60] Carnahan, Jill. "10 Health Tips For Anyone With A MTHFR Gene Mutation". Jill Carnahan, MD, 2014, https://www.jillcarnahan.com/2014/02/23/health-tips-for-anyone-with-a-mthfr-gene-mutation/. Accessed 19 Feb 2019.

[61] Jacobs, Elyn. "Iodine Deficiency: The Link Between Low Iodine & Cancer". The Truth About Cancer, 2019, https://thetruthaboutcancer.com/low-iodine-cancer/.

[62] Dyer, Diane. "Flaxseeds And Breast Cancer". Oncologynutrition.Org, 2014, https://www.oncologynutrition.org/erfc/healthy-nutrition-now/foods/flaxseeds-and-breast-cancer.

[63] Jacobs, Elyn. "The Truth About Estrogen And Breast Cancer". The Truth About Cancer, 2017, https://thetruthaboutcancer.com/estrogen-and-breast-cancer/.

[64] Horne, RH (AHG), Steven, and Kimberly Balas, ND. *The Comprehensive Guide To Nature's Sunshine Products*. 6th ed., Tree Of Light, 2014, p. 57.

[65] Rampton, John. "20 Quotes From Jim Rohn Putting Success And Life Into Perspective". *Entrepreneur*, 2016, https://www.entrepreneur.com/article/271873.

[66] "Smoking: What Are The Effects? - Mydr.Com.Au". *Mydr.Com.Au*, 2012, https://www.mydr.com.au/addictions/smoking-what-are-the-effects.

[67] "Xenoestrogens: What Are They, How To Avoid Them". *Women In Balance Institute*, 2012, https://womeninbalance.org/2012/10/26/xenoestrogens-what-are-they-how-to-avoid-them/.

[68] "Drinking Levels Defined | National Institute On Alcohol Abuse And Alcoholism (NIAAA)". *NIAAA.NIH.Gov*, https://www.niaaa.nih.gov/alcohol-health/overview-alcohol-consumption/moderate-binge-drinking.

[69] Frähm, David J. *A Cancer Battle Plan Sourcebook*. Penguin Putnam, 2000, p. 68.

[70] "Known And Probable Human Carcinogens". *Cancer.Org*, 2014, https://www.cancer.org/cancer/cancer-causes/general-info/known-and-probable-human-carcinogens.html.

[71] Horne, RH (AHG), Steven, and Kimberly Balas, ND. *The Comprehensive Guide To Nature's Sunshine Products*. 6th ed., Tree Of Light, 2014, pp. 56-59, 65, 113.

[72] "Exercise Linked With Lower Risk Of 13 Types Of Cancer". *Cancer.Org*, 2016, https://www.cancer.org/latest-news/exercise-linked-with-lower-risk-of-13-types-of-cancer.html.

[73] Howley, Elaine K. "How Does Sleep Influence Cancer Risk?". *US News*, 2018, https://health.usnews.com/health-care/patient-advice/articles/2018-07-04/how-does-sleep-influence-cancer-risk.

[74] Stevenson, Shawn. *Sleep Smarter: 21 Essential Strategies To Sleep Your Way To A Better Body, Better Health, And Bigger Success*. Rodale Inc., 2016, p. xxi.

[75] "How Much Sleep Do We Really Need? | National Sleep Foundation". *Sleepfoundation.Org*, https://www.sleepfoundation.org/excessive-sleepiness/support/how-much-sleep-do-we-really-need.

[76] "Psychological Stress And Cancer". *National Cancer Institute*, 2012, https://www.cancer.gov/about-cancer/coping/feelings/stress-fact-sheet

[77] Mandela, Nelson. "Lighting Your Way To A Better Future". 2003.

[78] Sparks, Nicholas. *The Notebook*. Warner Books, Inc., 1999, p. 5.

[79] "Funding For Research Areas". *National Cancer Institute*, 2018, https://www.cancer.gov/about-nci/budget/fact-book/data/research-funding.

Bibliography

Amen, Daniel G. *Change Your Brain, Change Your Life*. Harmony, 2015.

Barnard, Neal D, and Jennifer K Reilly. *The Cancer Survivor's Guide*. Healthy Living Publications, 2008.

Buttar, Rashid A. *The 9 Steps To Keep The Doctor Away*. Greenleaf Book Group Press, 2010.

Campbell, T. Colin, and Thomas M Campbell II. *The China Study: The Most Comprehensive Study Of Nutrition Ever Conducted And The Startling Implications For Diet, Weight Loss And Long-term Health*. BenBella Books, Inc., 2006.

Campbell, T. Colin, and Howard Jacobson. *Whole: Rethinking The Science Of Nutrition*. BenBella Books, Inc., 2013.

Carr, Kris. *Crazy Sexy Diet: Eat Your Veggies, Ignite Your Spark, And Live Like You Mean It!* Globe Pequot Press, 2011.

Esselstyn, Jr., Caldwell B. *Prevent And Reverse Heart Disease.* Avery, 2008.

"Famous Quotes At Brainyquote". *Brainyquote*, 2019, https://www.brainyquote.com.

Greger, Michael. *How Not To Die: Discover The Foods Scientifically Proven To Prevent And Reverse Disease.* FLATIRON Books, 2015.

McDougall, John A, and Mary A McDougall. *The Starch Solution: Eat The Foods You Love, Regain Your Health, And Lose The Weight For Good.* Rodale, 2012.

Somers, Suzanne. *Knockout: Interviews With Doctors Who Are Curing Cancer And How To Prevent Getting It In The First Place.* Three Rivers Press, 2010.

Stevenson, Shawn. *Sleep Smarter: 21 Essential Strategies To Sleep Your Way To A Better Body, Better Health, And Bigger Success.* Rodale Inc., 2016, p. xxi.

Wark, Chris. *Chris Beat Cancer.* Hay House, Inc., 2018.

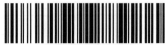

Made in the USA
Middletown, DE
31 March 2019